Sarvee Moosavi • Ali Rezaie
Nipaporn Pichetshote

Atlas of High-Resolution Manometry, Impedance, and pH Monitoring

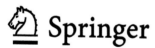

Springer

Sarvee Moosavi, MD, FRCPC
Department of Gastroenterology
and Hepatology
University of British Columbia
Vancouver, BC
Canada

Mark Pimentel, MD, FRCP(C)
Executive Director, Medically Associated
Science and Technology (MAST) Program
Cedars-Sinai Medical Center
Los Angeles, CA
USA

Ali Rezaie, MD, MSc, FRCPC
Cedars-Sinai Medical Center
Los Angeles, CA
USA

Nipaporn Pichetshote, MD
Cedars-Sinai Medical Center
Los Angeles, CA
USA

ISBN 978-3-030-27243-2   ISBN 978-3-030-27241-8   (eBook)
https://doi.org/10.1007/978-3-030-27241-8

This Springer imprint is published by the registered company Springer Nature Switzerland AG
The registered company address is: Gewerbestrasse 11, 6330 Cham, Switzerland

Preface

The field of gastrointestinal (GI) motility evaluation has been revolutionized over the past two decades with the advent of high-resolution manometry and impedance. The *Atlas of High-Resolution Manometry, Impedance, and pH Monitoring* is a unique, comprehensive reference book that allows the readers with various background knowledge to become familiar with the basic and advanced principles of GI motility assessment, specifically covering the manometry and pH monitoring in detail. Throughout the chapters, the readers are introduced to cases with increasing complexity. All slides come courtesy from the GI motility laboratory at Cedars-Sinai, Los Angeles, California. Compiled over the past decade, these slides provide the readers with a case-based discussion. Cases were selected from over 10,000 manometry and pH procedures, which were all performed and interpreted by the GI motility expert gastroenterologists.

The atlas portrays the realistic and pragmatic diagnostic capabilities of high-resolution manometry, impedance, and pH monitoring in day-to-day clinical practice. The first chapter includes the principles of esophageal manometry and impedance, while reviewing the study interpretation using the most currently available Chicago classification (version 3.0). It further discusses ways to troubleshoot the common challenges faced during these procedures. While standardization of basic components of manometry by the Chicago classification has significantly advanced the field, it does not cover impedance and numerous manometric/impedance findings associated with various diseases that are only detectable via "pattern recognition". Hence, the second chapter delves into cases beyond the Chicago classification. The third chapter covers the basic principles of antroduodenal manometry, a highly specialized motility test that is only available in a few centres around the world. Chapter four covers the intricacies of anorectal manometry. The final chapter is an updated review on the approach to "pH monitoring and impedance."

We hope this atlas provides a valuable and comprehensive resource for gastroenterologists, surgeons, residents, fellows motility nurses and GI motility lab techni-
cians around the world. Most importantly, we sincerely hope that the use of this
atlas will lead to improved care of our patients.

Vancouver, BC, Canada	Sarvee Moosavi
Los Angeles, CA, USA	Ali Rezaie
Los Angeles, CA, USA	Mark Pimentel
Los Angeles, CA, USA	Nipaporn Pichetshote

Contents

Chapter 1
Introduction to High-Resolution Manometry and Impedance

Gastrointestinal (GI) motility disorders are very common. Even though these conditions do not directly affect the life expectancy of the individuals, they certainly impact the quality of life and have both direct and indirect health-care costs. For patients with persistent severe symptoms despite routine therapies, investigations of GI motility may be warranted to further optimize care.

With the advent of various techniques for measuring intraluminal pressure events throughout the GI tract, the motor function of the gut is more easily assessed and its disorders are better understood. Systems for recording of intraluminal pressure events have evolved from simple balloons to water-perfused catheters and subsequently to solid-state catheters. Consequently, display and analysis methods have also evolved from strip chart conventional recording to computerized, high-resolution manometry (HRM) of seamless isobaric esophageal pressure topography (EPT). The perfused manometric system fell out of favor with the advent of HRM roughly 20 years ago, which provides a better description and further details of complex GI motility, while making it easier for the interpreter to analyze the data and further appreciate subtle findings that may have been overlooked with conventional manometry.

The Chicago Classification of esophageal manometry was developed to facilitate the interpretation of clinical HRM, thereby abandoning conventional manometry reporting. Hence, this atlas solely reviews all the aspects of HRM [1].

This introductory chapter reviews the fundamentals of HRM, including the technical aspects of esophageal HRM, indications, contraindications, safety, and tolerability, as well as the basics of interpreting a study. Chapter 2 delves into details of esophageal manometry and discusses the diagnostic criteria of various esophageal motility disorders [1].

It is critical to use the descriptive part of the chapter along with the supplemental illustrations throughout each section to better understand the principles of interpretation of manometry studies.

© Springer Nature Switzerland AG 2020
S. Moosavi et al., *Atlas of High-Resolution Manometry, Impedance, and pH Monitoring*, https://doi.org/10.1007/978-3-030-27241-8_1

Overview: High-Resolution Manometry: How Does It Work?

Advances in both hardware and software technology have made high-resolution manometry recording possible. Each HRM catheter contains 36 sensors, spaced 1 cm apart longitudinally and radially, spanning a length of 35 cm (Fig. 1.1). Each sensor measures pressure from 12 positions in its circumference and averages out these measurements. In the esophagus, this allows simultaneous recording from the proximal pharynx, upper esophageal sphincter, esophageal body, lower esophageal sphincter, and proximal stomach without repositioning the catheter, as was formerly required with conventional water-perfused manometry.

The software allows the pressure data to be analyzed simultaneously as it is displayed by color contours corresponding to various intraluminal pressures. In an esophageal pressure topography, the data is outlined in spatiotemporal plots, with location and time recorded as continuous variables on the X and Y axes, respectively. The pressure magnitude is shown at each x-y coordinate by color. As seen in Figure 1.2, lower pressures are shown as cold colors and higher pressures are depicted as hot colors. Isobaric contours are pressure lines that are used to outline the locations where the pressure is the same in the color contour plot on HRM (Fig. 1.3). The reader can change the gain (i.e., the pressure-color relationship) to appreciate further details (Fig. 1.4).

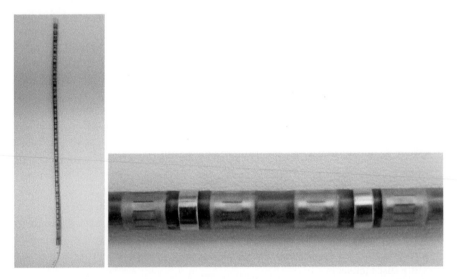

Figure 1.1 Solid-state catheter for high-resolution esophageal manometry with impedance. As seen in the closeup image, the pressure sensors are interspersed with the impedance catheters. The pressure sensors allow the measurement of circumferential pressure along the length of the esophagus. These catheters are quite delicate and should be handled with care to avoid damaging the sensors or the catheter sheath

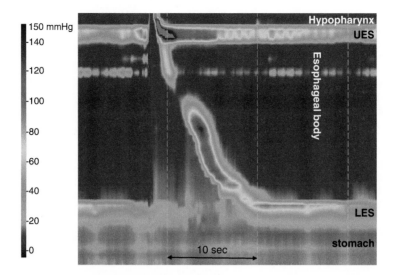

Figure 1.2 High-resolution esophageal manometry of a normal wet swallow. The high-resolution esophageal manometry catheter allows simultaneous measurement of the pressures from the hypopharynx, the upper esophageal sphincter (UES), the esophageal body, the lower esophageal sphincter (LES), and the proximal stomach. The high-pressure zones are depicted as "hotter" colors, while the lower-pressure zones are shown as "cooler" colors. The color-pressure reference bar is seen on the left side

While this brief introduction to the technique of HRM has focused on the esophagus, the same basic principles equally apply to recordings from other segments of the GI tract, including antroduodenal and anorectal manometry. The HRM color contour pressure plot provides an array of numeric data, which allows the reader to develop the skillset for pattern recognition of common GI motility disorders. This will be reviewed in depth throughout this atlas.

Technique

The technique for insertion of an esophageal manometric catheter is similar to that of nasogastric tube insertion. The patient is placed comfortably in a semi-supine position. Usually, a topical anesthetic such as lidocaine 2% is used intranasally. This is preferably applied as a gel by a cotton swab rather than in spray form, which may increase the risk of aspiration. The catheter is then slowly advanced intranasally. The patient can be asked to tilt his or her head forward, tucking the chin to the chest to facilitate catheter advancement. Once the catheter reaches the upper esophageal sphincter, the technician or gastroenterologist may feel a slight resistance. In addition, a high-pressure zone may be seen on the screen (Fig. 1.5). The subject is then asked to take small sips of water to facilitate catheter advancement in the body of the esophagus. A second high-pressure zone is seen on the screen, which is the

Figure 1.3 High-resolution esophageal manometry with various isobaric pressure contours. Isobaric contour lines (*black lines*) can be set up at various pressures to outline the area of interest. These figures show isobaric pressure set at 20 mm Hg (**A**), 30 mm Hg (**B**), and 40 mm Hg (**C**). The inner area outlined by isobaric lines shows the locations on the esophageal pressure-color plots with pressure equal to or greater than that of the related isobaric contour lines. The area outside of the isobaric contour lines has pressure lower than that of the isobaric line

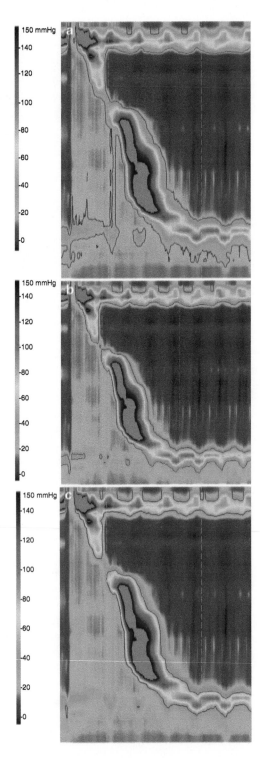

Figure 1.4 High-resolution esophageal manometry of various pressure amplification of the color-pressure topography. A, The magenta color (*asterisk*) represents pressures out of the maximum set range. The higher-pressure amplitude can be brought within the range by increasing the maximum on the pressure range, and low-amplitude pressure events can be brought into range by decreasing the minimum on the pressure range. The pressure range for each manometry is shown to the left of the manometry figure. In **A,** the pressure range is set up at -10 mm Hg to 150 mm Hg. **B,** The maximum pressure zone is increased to 200 mm Hg, which leads to a decrease in the area out of the pressure range

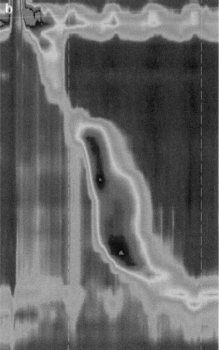

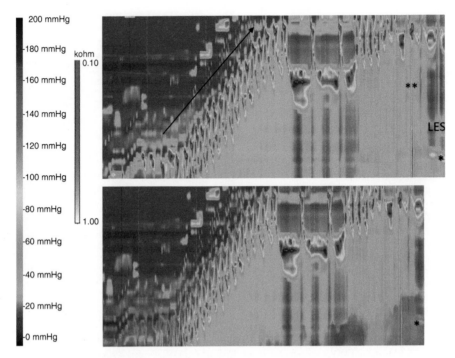

Figure 1.5 High-resolution esophageal manometry of catheter insertion. The **top** tracing shows advancement of the esophageal manometry catheter through the hypopharynx (*arrow*). The UES contour is seen with intermittent relaxation upon wet swallows. The patient had an episode of gag (*double asterisks*), demonstrated by column of pressure originating from the stomach. The patient is ultimately asked to take a deep breath, which causes diaphragmatic contraction (*asterisk*). This allows the technician or gastroenterologist to recognize that the catheter has traversed the diaphragm. There appears to be a small sliding hiatal hernia, as the LES resting pressure is separated from the diaphragmatic contraction. The **bottom** image shows the same tracing with impedance. The impedance is decreased as the catheter is passed through the nasopharynx, owing to the electrolyte-rich secretion in the nasal cavities. The salt water entered the stomach. There is some hold-up in the hiatal hernia sac

lower esophageal sphincter. To verify whether the catheter has traversed the diaphragm and entered the stomach, the subject is asked to take a deep breath in and out, to identify the pressure variation cycles in the thoracic and abdominal cavities, as well as the diaphragmatic crural contraction during inspiration. This stage is further reviewed in Chapter 2, under "Pressure Inversion Point."

The study is started by recording 30 seconds of "rest" as the subject sits calmly, breathes quietly, and avoids swallowing. The landmark recording is documented after pushing the "start" button on the software and is automatically concluded at the end of 30 seconds. Subsequently, each wet swallow with 5 mL of normal saline is initiated with pushing the "start" button. Each swallow should be recorded for at least 20 uninterrupted seconds. If the patient swallows prematurely during this interval or double swallows (Fig. 1.6), the recording of that particular swallow should be reset and recorded again. A total of 10 wet swallows

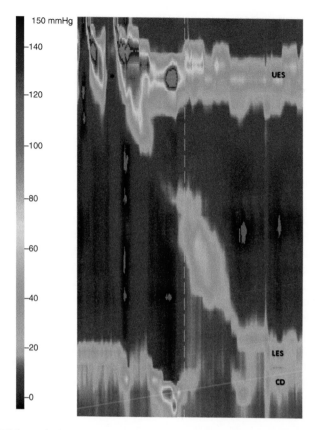

Figure 1.6 High-resolution esophageal manometry of a "double swallow." Patients are asked to take 10 swallows during HRM data acquisition, but sometimes patients may take two consecutive swallows. This image shows an example of a "double swallow," where two consecutive relaxations in the upper esophageal resting pressure are noted, with the first one initiated with the onset of the wet swallow. The second relaxation corresponds to a dry swallow, or double swallow. As the second swallow occurred shortly after the first one, the first swallow was inhibited and did not result in a peristaltic contraction. The second swallow (*asterisk*) resulted in a peristaltic contraction. In this case, the swallow should be repeated during the data acquisition. Note that the crural diaphragm (CD) is roughly 2 cm distal to the LES, indicating a 2-cm hiatal hernia

with liquid (i.e. normal saline) is obtained. Some centers routinely obtain viscous swallows as well. It is also possible to obtain wet swallows in response to a solid bolus, but no reference range or unified test substance is yet reported in the consensus. Therefore, throughout this atlas, the normal values are reported for a clear liquid bolus.

Once the study is concluded, the catheter is pulled and is suspended in the air ex-vivo, without touching the sensors. This step is crucial for equilibrating the catheter and eliminating the background noise later. At the end of the study, thermal compensation should be performed through the software to eliminate background noise and allow appropriate interpretation of the study.

Safety and Tolerability

Esophageal manometry is generally considered a safe procedure. In a study by Huang et al. [2], esophageal manometry was shown to be safe and well-tolerated. Serious complications were very rare (0.1%), including self-limited hypertension and hypoxia. The rate of incomplete procedure due to intolerability and difficult insertion is low, at roughly 4%.

Indications and Contraindications

The most common indication for esophageal HRM is to further evaluate non-obstructive dysphagia in subjects with persistent symptoms (Table 1.1). It is note-worthy to mention that the endoscopist may appreciate esophageal dysmotility along the body of the esophagus or the absence of appropriate lower esophageal sphincter relaxation at the time of the upper endoscopy, which could be suggestive of achalasia or other esophagogastric junction outflow obstruction. However, upper endoscopy has very low sensitivity to identify any esophageal dysmotility disorders; therefore further characterization of these disorders requires esophageal manometry. In addition, the endoscopists should use clinical acumen to decide whether any other ancillary investigations such as chest x-ray or CT scan are required before arranging esophageal HRM. Further details on the workup of dysphagia are outside the scope of this atlas.

Table 1.1 High-Resolution Esophageal Manometry: Indications and Contraindications

Indications
Non-obstructive dysphagia of unclear etiology
Query diagnosis of esophagogastric junction outflow obstruction, especially achalasia
Query diagnosis of impaired esophageal motility and/or abnormal bolus clearance (e.g. connective tissue disorder, scleroderma)
Preoperative evaluation for antireflux surgery, for objective assessment of esophagogastric junction subtypes and contractility
Assessment of recurrent symptoms after antireflux surgery or other esophageal interventions for major motility disorders (e.g. Per oral endoscopic myotomy [POEM])
Accurate placement of pH-monitoring catheter
Emerging role in upper esophageal sphincter abnormality and oropharyngeal dysphagia
Emerging role in patients with interstitial lung disease and in preoperative assessment of patients undergoing lung transplantation, such as scleroderma
Contraindications
Decreased level of consciousness
Inability to follow instructions because of cognitive, mental, or language barrier
Basal skull fracture or recent nasal fracture

Other common situations that may warrant esophageal manometry include non-cardiac chest pain, gastroesophageal reflux disease (with or without subsequent pH monitoring, which requires HRM for proper pH catheter placement), and systemic diseases affecting striated or smooth muscles of the esophagus or the autonomic nervous system. Subjects undergoing surgical management of hiatal hernia also require esophageal HRM preoperatively to further characterize the integrity of the esophagogastric junction, to accurately estimate the size of the hiatal hernia, and to assess the "esophageal peristaltic reserve," which is shown to be a pre-operative factor predicting whether late postoperative dysphagia may develop (beyond 3 months) [3].

Absolute contraindications to HRM are rare. These include decreased level of consciousness, basal skull, or recent nasal fracture. In subjects with remote nasal fracture, surgery, or septal deviation, HRM catheter insertion may be challenging. In these circumstances, if there is no contraindication, both nares should be attempted for manometry catheter insertion. Topical lidocaine in nasal passages could be used to alleviate discomfort and improve tolerability. The subject should be alert and able to follow instruction during catheter insertion. Caution should be practiced when performing HRM on subjects with oropharyngeal dysphagia and supressed cough reflex, especially when the subject is asked to swallow sips of water to advance the catheter. This maneuver could potentially increase the risk of aspiration. Finally, HRM is generally safely done in subjects on oral anticoagulation, including warfarin or novel oral anticoagulant agents. Therefore, these agents are generally not interrupted for esophageal HRM. Rare complications such as mild epistaxis or sore throat could occur, which is usually self-limited. If the subject coughs persistently during catheter insertion, advancement of the catheter should be stopped. The catheter should be pulled back, to ensure that it is not in the trachea or folded in the hypopharynx. Other chapters will review further insertion tips.

High-Resolution Manometry Protocol

The subject should fast for 4–5 hours prior to HRM, primarily to avoid aspiration due to vomiting. The operator reviews the details of the HRM procedure with the subject before inserting the HRM catheter. To increase tolerability of catheter insertion during the HRM study, topical anesthetic with lidocaine 2% gel is often used in the nares. Some centers may use lidocaine spray in the oropharynx, but this could theoretically impact the hypopharynx and upper esophageal motility, so its regular use is not advised. The operator should review the list of subject's medications, as many agents could impact the esophageal motility, particularly opioids.

The subject sits quietly in an upright position. HRM catheter is inserted intra-nasally, and is advanced slowly, while the technician or the physician follows the pressure topography color contour to recognize upper (UES) and lower esophageal sphincters (LES) and ensures the catheter has traversed the LES into the proximal stomach. Once the HRM catheter is in the correct position, it does not

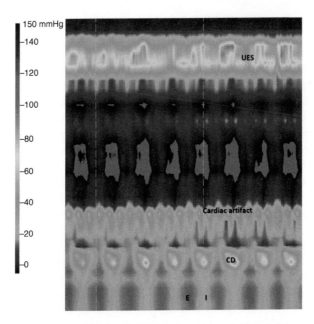

Figure 1.7 High-resolution esophageal manometry at rest. During the data acquisition, the patient is asked to remain calm for 30 seconds and avoid swallowing. In this HRM, there is a pulsatile, high-pressure zone that appears to repeat itself at a rate faster than respiration. This corresponds to a cardiac or vasculature artifact. This finding may be normal, due to proximity of the esophagus to the right atrium, right ventricle, and aorta. Vascular artifacts on esophageal manometry may be also seen in a setting of aberrant aortic branches or cardiomegaly. The crural diaphragm (CD) is recognized easily, as it contracts with inspiration. The pressure respiratory variation is marked with E (expiration) and I (inspiration)

require repositioning. The technician is then asked to hold the catheter in place or gently tape the catheter to the nasal bridge to avoid any displacement during the manometry study.

During the HRM study, the subject is asked to remain calm and avoid swallowing for 30 seconds for landmark measurements, to help determine resting LES and UES pressures (Fig. 1.7). The subject then undergoes a 10-swallow protocol, consisting of 10 wet swallows, each with 5 mL normal saline. As mentioned previously, although other provocative swallows with viscous or solid food could be added to the protocol, currently there are few validated metrics to determine the significance of swallow patterns seen with these substances.

Impedance

Impedance is essentially defined as resistance to electrical flow or other forms of energy, labelled as symbol Z on HRM studies. As demonstrated in Figures 1.2 and 1.8, air has the highest impedance (i.e., lowest electrical conductivity) and refluxate

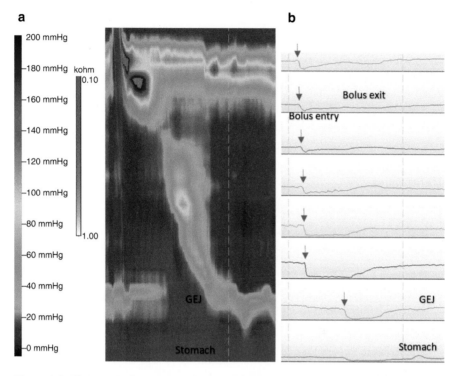

Figure 1.8 High-resolution manometry with impedance. A, A normal wet swallow response. The UES opens normally. The impedance is seen as the purple hue. The impedance drops with salt water, as the electrolytes allow electrical conductivity. Once the bolus clears the esophagus (deeper purple), the impedance returns to the baseline. **B,** Impedance readings on line setting. The impedance drops sequentially below a 50% threshold upon bolus entry (*arrows*). Ultimately, the impedance returns to its baseline and remains above the threshold, which suggests that the bolus completely clears the esophagus. Note that no significant drop is seen in the stomach because of its continuous low impedance

and food have the lowest impedance (i.e., highest electrical conductivity) because of the presence of electrolytes. Thus, saline swallows are used to maximize impedance measures.

Impedance has become an integral and complementary part of HRM, as multi-channel intraluminal impedance has allowed evaluation of bolus transit without radiation. Catheters for HRM with impedance generally have 16 impedance sensors at 2-cm intervals, interspersed with 36 circumferential pressure sensors. In this way, impedance can be assessed at the same time as the pressure measurements. Upon bolus entry (e.g., 5 mL of normal saline on wet swallow), the intraluminal esophageal impedance drops below the baseline and remains low until the bolus exits the esophagus. In a study by Cho et al. [4], the bolus entry was defined as a decrease in impedance by more than 50% of baseline, and bolus exit was defined as the return to the value that defined entry. Swallows were classified as "complete bolus transit" if bolus entry occurred at the most proximal site (20 cm above the LES) and bolus exit points were recorded for all three distal sites at which impedance was measured (i.e. at 15, 10, and 5 cm above the LES). Therefore, bolus passage manifests as a 50% drop in impedance and an eventual return to baseline. This technique has been validated with a 97% concordance in the assessment of esophageal emptying in healthy subjects undergoing videofluoroscopy [5, 6]. Of note, the assessment of impedance is not covered by the Chicago Classification of esophageal motility disorders.

The examples of HRM and impedance throughout this atlas have been obtained using a Medtronic manometry system.

References

1. Kahrilas PJ, Bredenoord AJ, Fox M, Gyawali CP, Roman S, Smout AJ, Pandolfino JE, International High Resolution Manometry Working Group. The Chicago Classification of esophageal motility disorders, v3.0. Neurogastroenterol Motil. 2015;27:160–74.
2. Huang L, Hom C, Chen T, Pimentel M, Rezaie A. Safety and tolerability of high-resolution esophageal manometry: a large database analysis [Abstract]. Gastroenterology. 2017;152(5, Suppl 1):S325.
3. Shaker A, Stoikes N, Drapekin J, Kushnir V, Brunt LM, Gyawali CP. Multiple rapid swallow responses during esophageal high-resolution manometry reflect esophageal body peristaltic reserve. Am J Gastroenterol. 2013;108:1706–12.
4. Cho YK, Choi MG, Oh SN, Baik CN, Park JM, Lee IS, et al. Comparison of bolus transit patterns identified by esophageal impedance to barium esophagram in patients with dysphagia. Dis Esophagus. 2012;25:17–25.
5. Simrén M, Silny J, Holloway R, Tack J, Janssens J, Sifrim D. Relevance of ineffective oesophageal motility during oesophageal acid clearance. Gut. 2003;52:784–90.
6. Imam H, Shay S, Ali A, Baker M. Bolus transit patterns in healthy subjects: a study using simultaneous impedance monitoring, videoesophagram, and esophageal manometry. Am J Physiol Gastrointest Liver Physiol. 2005;288:G1000–6.

Chapter 2
Esophageal Manometry

This chapter discusses in detail the normal manometric landmarks, with the text describing the principles behind these landmarks and the illustrations serving as a reference for using the concepts and applying them to esophageal manometry studies. Throughout this chapter (unless stated otherwise), each swallow on esophageal pressure topography (EPT) should be considered to be 10 seconds in duration, as shown in Figure 2.1, which demonstrates one normal wet swallow. This is applicable throughout the chapter, unless it is stated otherwise per illustration. The color chart on the left side of the illustration represents the pressure plot.

Impedance is highlighted in Figure 2.2. On the left side appears an additional bar of various purple color tones, with darker purple showing lower impedance (i.e., higher electrical conductivity between two adjacent impedance sensors).

Normal High-Resolution Esophageal Manometry

Upper Esophageal Sphincter

The first resting esophageal landmark is the upper esophageal sphincter (UES), a musculature closure composed mainly of the cricopharyngeus muscle but also including the inferior pharyngeal muscle and cervical esophagus. The UES opens with the onset of a swallow, but it can also open intermittently to allow transsphincteric flow of gas or fluid for esophageal venting or belching. The primary function of the UES is to prevent air insufflation of the esophagus during inspiration, when the intrathoracic pressure becomes negative. It also protects the hypopharynx from retrograde movement of gastric contents.

© Springer Nature Switzerland AG 2020
S. Moosavi et al., *Atlas of High-Resolution Manometry, Impedance, and pH Monitoring*, https://doi.org/10.1007/978-3-030-27241-8_2

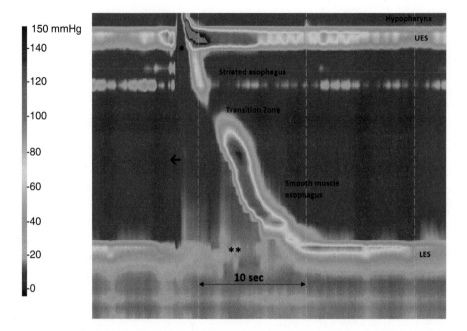

Figure 2.1   High-resolution manometry (HRM) of normal esophageal peristalsis. The HRM catheter is inserted in the esophagus and traverses the lower esophageal sphincter (LES) into the stomach. This technique allows simultaneous pressure recordings of the hypopharynx, upper esophageal sphincter (UES), esophagus, LES, and stomach. The sensor location is on the y-axis; the x-axis is time. The color contour demonstrates the pressure recordings along the length of the catheter at a given time and location. The resting UES pressure is shown as a horizontal color band, several few centimeters wide, with pressures greater than the adjacent pharynx. The resting LES pressure is also seen as a horizontal color band in the distal esophagus, with resting pressure greater than that of the adjacent esophagus and stomach. The relaxations of the UES (*asterisk*) and LES (*double asterisks*) are shown as decreases in pressures, demonstrated as changes in color to teal (corresponding to approximately 20 mm Hg on color-pressure bar). The UES relaxation pressure (*asterisk*) approximates that of the proximal esophagus, and the LES relaxation pressure (*double asterisks*) approximates that of the stomach. The LES opens shortly after the UES relaxation with the onset of the wet swallow. Esophageal primary peristalsis is shown as a diagonal color band running from the UES to the LES. HRM shows the high-pressure contraction in the proximal, striated esophagus, followed by a lower-pressure segment corresponding to the transition zone, and a subsequent increase in pressure in the smooth muscle esophagus. Intrabolus pressure (*arrow*)—that is, pressure in the swallowed bolus—is represented by a small simultaneous rise in intraesophageal pressure. It occurs shortly after the beginning of the wet swallow and remains elevated ahead of the peristaltic pressure wave. This pressure returns back to baseline after the peristaltic wave passes, indicating the bolus clearance from the esophagus

As seen in Figure 2.1, the UES is seen on esophageal manometry as a horizontal band of high pressure proximally. With the onset of swallow, the UES pressure decreases and approximates the proximal esophageal pressure. After the bolus passes, the UES pressure returns to baseline.

Low UES pressure (UES hypotension) can be seen in patients with skeletal muscle pathology, including myasthenia gravis and muscular dystrophy, or

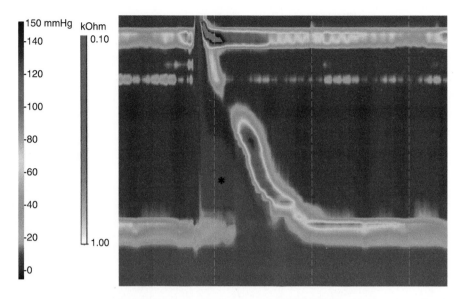

Figure 2.2 High-resolution esophageal manometry with impedance of a wet swallow.
Impedance is a measurement of resistance to electrical conductivity. Normal saline contains electrolytes (Na+ and Cl−), which allow electrical conduction, identified by two adjacent impedance sensors at any point along the manometry/impedance catheter. Impedance is inversely proportional to conductivity: fluid has the lowest conductivity, while air has the highest conductivity. The purple hue (∗) shows low impedance, due to presence of normal saline. With the onset of the wet swallow, the fluid is propagated by primary peristalsis and subsequently enters the stomach. With LES pressure returning to its baseline at the end of the wet swallow, there is no residual fluid bolus in the esophagus. Therefore, the bolus has completely cleared the esophagus, and the impedance returns to its baseline

neurodegenerative diseases such as Parkinson's disease or stroke. In addition, head and neck radiation therapy can cause UES hypotension.

On the contrary, UES hypertension can also occur during esophageal manometry. This is most often caused by the catheter irritation of hypopharynx and patient's anxiety. However, several possible differential diagnoses should be considered:

- Cricopharyngeal bar
- Proximal esophageal web or rings
- Cervical osteophytes or orthopedic cervical metal plates
- Massive thyromegaly
- Zenker's diverticulum
- Secondary manifestation of impaired lower esophageal sphincter (LES) relaxation: achalasia, esophagogastric junction outflow obstruction

Figure 2.3 demonstrates high-resolution manometry (HRM) findings of UES hypotension and hypertension.

Figure 2.4 illustrates the normal action of the UES during swallowing.

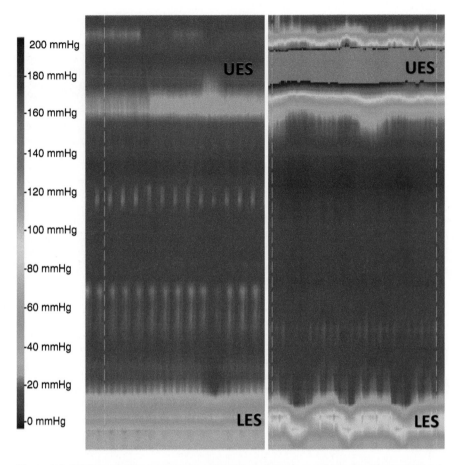

Figure 2.3 High-resolution manometry of upper and lower esophageal sphincters at rest. **Left,** A hypotensive upper esophageal sphincter (UES) with resting UES pressure approaching 0 mm Hg; the resting pressure of the lower esophageal sphincter (LES) is normal. The subject is at increased risk of aspiration. The differential diagnosis includes skeletal muscle disorders, head and neck radiation, stroke, or neurodegenerative diseases such as Parkinson's disease. **Right,** A hypertensive UES with resting pressure greater than 200 mm Hg and normal LES resting pressure. The most common differential diagnosis for a hypertensive UES is anxiety and hypopharyngeal irritation due to the manometry catheter. More rare causes include a cricopharyngeal bar, cervical osteophytes, massive thyromegaly, Zenker's diverticulum, and cricopharyngeal achalasia

Transition Zone

As demonstrated on a normal esophageal manometry in Figure 2.1, the transition zone is a small gap of low pressure between the proximal striated esophagus and the distal two thirds of the esophageal body. Composed of smooth muscles, it is believed to be an area of segmental contraction, which requires coordinated contractions of upper and lower esophageal waves for complete bolus clearance. However, its exact

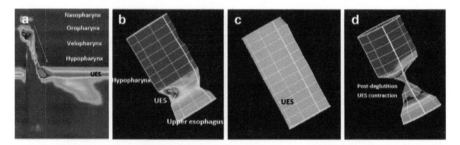

Figure 2.4 High-resolution esophageal manometry of the hypopharynx and the proximal esophagus during a wet swallow. A, With the onset of the wet swallow, the soft palate (velopharynx) rises, and with the contraction of base of the tongue, mesopharynx, and hypopharynx, the bolus is transferred towards the UES. This contraction results in a diagonal band of pressure (*arrow*) proximal to the UES. Subsequently, the UES opens and the bolus is transferred to the proximal striated esophagus, where the peristaltic contraction is initiated. The other three images show three-dimensional (3-D) esophageal manometry of the hypopharynx and UES, a technique that is limited to clinical research because of the fragility of the 3-D HRM catheter. **B,** A higher-pressure zone is seen around the UES at the bottom of the 3-D cylinder. Note that the UES is not symmetrical, as demonstrated by the variable pressure along its circumference. **C,** With the bolus transfer through the UES, the sphincter relaxes, and pressure of the UES approximates the proximal esophageal pressure. **D,** Once the bolus traverses through the UES, the sphincter closes, generating higher pressure to prevent aspiration

physiologic role is unclear. The transition zone may be effaced in subjects with a short esophagus or in the setting of anatomical abnormalities such as massive sliding hiatal hernia, as demonstrated in Figure 2.5.

Pressure Inversion Point (PIP)

On esophageal manometry, the pressure variation in the thoracic and abdominal cavities is easily appreciated during respiratory cycles. In the thoracic cavity, the pressure becomes negative on inspiration and positive on expiration. The pressure pattern is opposite in the intra-abdominal cavity. These two cavities are separated by the diaphragm. The pressure inversion point (PIP) is the landmark at which the pressure patterns above and below are the opposite of each other. This point most often coincides with the crural diaphragm which is more easily appreciated on deep inspiration.

On esophageal manometry in normal subjects, the LES and the crural diaphragm are closely juxtaposed. Therefore, the PIP is along the high-pressure zone composed of both the LES and crural diaphragm (Fig. 2.6). In different subtypes of esophagogastric junctions, however, PIP landmarks can vary, as detailed later. For example, in patients with sliding hiatal hernia, the LES and crural diaphragm are separated from each other, with the LES displaced into the thoracic cavity and the PIP along the crural diaphragm. On manometry, the size of the hiatal hernia can be accurately assessed by evaluating the distance between the PIP and LES.

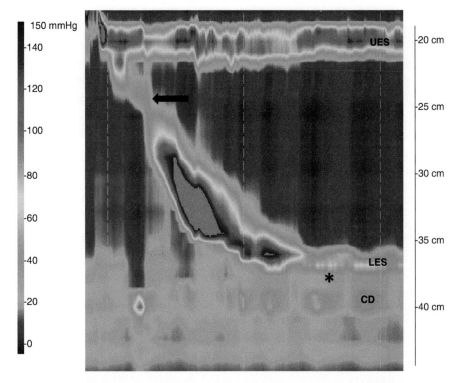

Figure 2.5   High-resolution manometry of a shortened esophagus with sliding hiatal hernia. The catheter length is marked on the right side. As demonstrated, the esophagus is shortened to 17 cm in length. The transition zone is obliterated (*arrow*). There is a 3-cm sliding hiatal hernia. Successful repair of the hiatal hernia in this patient will require both Nissen fundoplication and Collis gastroplasty, a procedure to lengthen the esophagus in order to prevent premature rupture of the Nissen band due to the pulling pressure of the shortened esophagus. Another phenomenon that can be observed in shortened esophagus is a falsely low contraction vigor, but the contraction vigor in this example is normal; the distal contractile integral (DCI) is greater than 450 mmHg.sec.cm

Lower Esophageal Sphincter

The next resting esophageal landmark is the lower esophageal sphincter (LES), a specialized segment of the circular muscularis propria of the distal esophagus that generates 90% of the resting pressure at the esophagogastric junction in normal subjects. It is usually 2–4 cm in length. The phrenoesophageal ligament holds the diaphragmatic crura in close proximity to the esophagogastric mucosal junction. Along with the crural diaphragm (CD), the LES generates a high-pressure zone in the distal esophagus, which serves as a barrier to gastric or bile reflux. Because the LES is closely related to the diaphragm, its contour moves with respiration. During inspiration, the diaphragm flattens, so the LES moves down. During expiration, the diaphragm relaxes and the LES moves up.

The LES is innervated by excitatory myenteric neurons secreting acetylcholine; the inhibitory neurons are nitrergic, secreting nitric oxide or vasoactive intestinal peptide (VIP), causing LES relaxation.

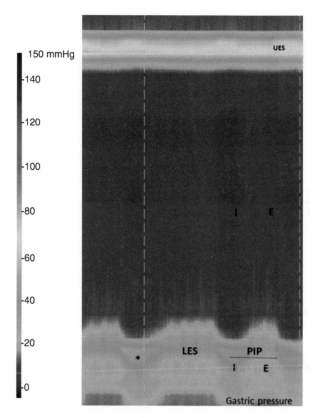

Figure 2.6 High-resolution manometry of the esophagus at rest: The pressure inversion point (PIP). The UES is seen as a horizontal band of pressure proximally, and the LES is seen distally. At the gastro-esophageal junction, the LES and crural diaphragm normally juxtapose and generate a high-pressure zone. The pattern of respiratory pressure variations differs between the thoracic and abdominal cavities. In the thoracic cavity (i.e., esophageal body), the pressure becomes more negative (darker blue) during inspiration (I), and more positive (lighter blue) with expiration (E). In the abdominal cavity, the cycle is reversed, with the pressure becoming more positive with inspiration owing to the flattening and contraction (*asterisk*) of the diaphragm, and more negative on expiration. This principle can be used during HRM to ensure that the catheter has traversed the diaphragm into the stomach. The pressure inversion point (PIP) is a landmark at which the respiratory variations in pressure cycles reverse, as described above. Following the above pattern, the PIP in this example is found to be along the LES

On esophageal manometry, the LES is seen as a high-pressure zone under tonic contraction in the distal esophagus. During the esophageal manometry data analysis, the upper and lower borders of the distal esophageal high-pressure zone in the "landmark" phase of the study are highlighted by placing the software markers along the appropriate margins. The LES pressure is measured relative to the gastric pressure. Therefore, the marker for the gastric pressure is placed in a "quiet" area with the lowest pressure, no contraction, and distal to the LES (Fig. 2.7). The software then calculates the LES pressure. If there is a hiatal hernia, as depicted by the separation between the LES high-pressure zone and crural diaphragmatic contractions, the LES borders excluding the hiatal hernia should be marked to accurately measure the LES pressure.

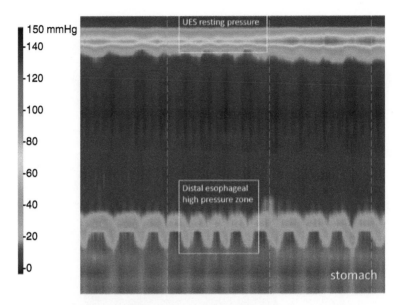

Figure 2.7 High-resolution esophageal manometry of resting pressures. During study acquisition, the patient is asked to remain calm and avoid swallowing for 30 seconds in order to obtain the resting pressure of the UES and the distal esophageal high-pressure zone (HPZ, composed of the LES and crural diaphragm). The software calculates the LES pressure relative to the gastric pressure. Therefore, the pressure cursor for the LES should be placed in the area with the highest pressure along the HPZ, and the pressure cursor for the stomach should be placed distal to the HPZ, in the area with lowest pressure

Normal basal LES pressure ranges from 4 to 32 mm Hg. The LES relaxes in response to the onset of the swallow, coinciding with UES relaxation. LES relaxation pressure usually approximates the proximal gastric pressure in normal subjects. This allows the bolus to pass through the LES ahead of the esophageal peristalsis. The LES then contracts strongly, once the peristaltic wave passes, to prevent reflux of gastric contents (Fig. 2.8).

Esophagogastric Junction (EGJ)

The final resting landmark is the esophagogastric junction (EGJ). Morphology has been shown to be important in determining EGJ barrier function, as separation between the LES and crural diaphragm (CD) facilitates reflux. In the Chicago Classification of esophageal motility disorders [1], three subtypes of EGJ are described, based on HRM and spatial pressure variation plots. In Type I EGJ (Fig. 2.9) corresponds to close juxtaposition of the LES and CD. Therefore, the PIP lies near the proximal margin of the EGJ. In Type II (Fig. 2.10), the EGJ has two peaks on the instantaneous spatial pressure variation plot; the nadir pressure is

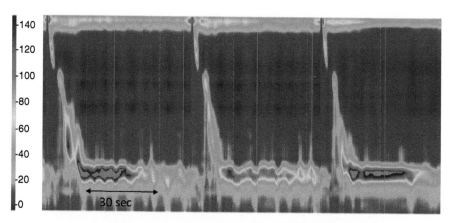

Figure 2.8 High-resolution esophageal manometry of lower esophageal sphincter spasm. Shown are three wet swallows that resulted in normal primary peristalsis. After wet swallows, the LES pressure is elevated up to 150 mm Hg, as shown by the red hue along the LES pressure zone. The spasm lasts approximately 40 seconds. The LES relaxes normally, so this HRM illustration does not meet criteria for esophagogastric junction outflow obstruction. The significance of this finding is unclear, but when it is seen, wet swallows should be spaced out to avoid a false increase in integrated relaxation pressure (IRP) of the LES

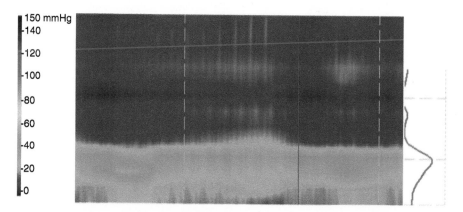

Figure 2.9 High-resolution esophageal manometry of Type I esophagogastric junction (EGJ). The instantaneous spatial pressure variation plot is shown on the right side. It represents the pressure plot, noted where the vertical red line is placed on the HRM. This pressure plot shows one peak. The two components of the EGJ are the LES and CD. In a Type I EGJ, these two components are superimposed. The pressure inversion point (PIP) lies near the proximal margin of the EGJ. During inspiration, the EGJ pressure increases, whereas it decreases during expiration

greater than the intragastric pressure, and the separation distance between the LES and CD is 1–2 cm. Finally, in Type III, the EGJ has two peaks on the instantaneous spatial pressure variation plot; the nadir pressure is equal to or lower than the intragastric pressure, and the separation between the LES and CD is greater than 2 cm. Type III is divided into two categories: In subtype IIIa (Fig. 2.11), the PIP is at the

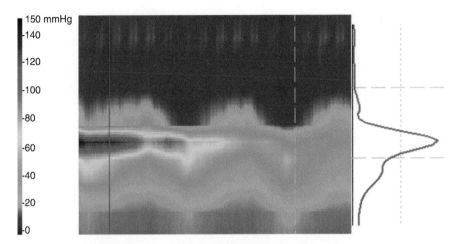

Figure 2.10 High-resolution esophageal manometry of Type II EGJ. The instantaneous spatial pressure variation plot is shown on the right side. It represents the pressure plot, noted where the vertical red line is placed on the HRM. This pressure plot shows two peaks, with the first one at the LES and the second one at the crural diaphragm (CD). The PIP is at the level of the CD. The nadir between the LES and the CD peaks is greater than the gastric pressure

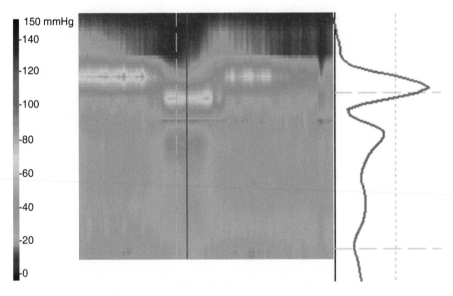

Figure 2.11 High-resolution esophageal manometry of Type IIIa EGJ. The instantaneous spatial pressure variation plot is shown on the right side. It represents the pressure plot, noted where the vertical red line is placed on the HRM. This pressure plot shows two peaks, with the first one at the LES and the second one at the CD. The PIP is at the level of the CD. The nadir between the LES and the CD peaks is equal to or less than the gastric pressure

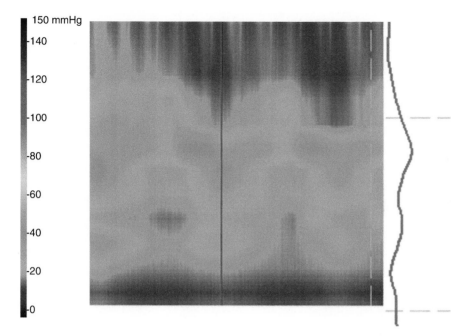

Figure 2.12 High-resolution esophageal manometry of type IIIb Esophagogastric junction.
The instantaneous spatial pressure variation plot is shown on the right side. It represents the pressure plot, noted where the vertical red line is placed on the HRM. This pressure plot shows two
peaks, with the first one at the LES and the second one at the CD. The PIP is at the level of the
LES. The nadir between the LES and the CD peaks is equal to the gastric pressure. With a type IIIb
EGJ, the nadir between the LES and the CD peaks also can be less than the gastric pressure. The
pressure variation between the LES and the CD with respiration follows the opposite pattern to that
of the intrathoracic cavity

CD level, whereas in subtype IIIb (Fig. 2.12), the PIP is at the LES. In a double-
peak pattern, the separation distance between CD and LES is reported as the axial
distance between the two peaks.

Length of Esophagus

Contractile Segments

On normal esophageal manometry, there are two contractile segments. The upper
third of the esophagus is composed of striated esophagus. The contraction in striated
esophagus is seen as the first segment of peristalsis, proximal to the transition zone.
The contraction is mediated by sequential excitation of lower motor neurons mediated
by the vagus nerve from the nucleus ambiguus. The middle third of the esophagus has

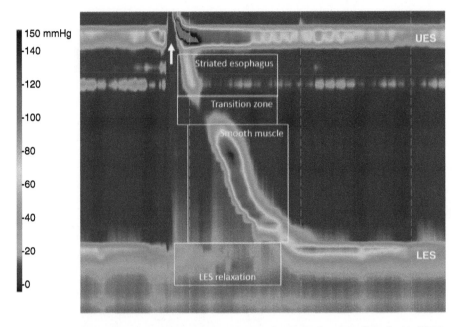

Figure 2.13 High-resolution esophageal manometry of a normal wet swallow. In this HRM, the two contractile segments of the esophagus are highlighted. With the onset of the wet swallow, the UES relaxes (*arrow*), and the primary peristaltic contraction ensues. The onset of LES relaxation also coincides with the onset of the wet swallow

a mixture of skeletal and smooth muscle fibers; the distal third is composed solely of smooth muscle. The second and third contractile segments are seen distal to the transition zone on the high-resolution esophageal manometry (Fig. 2.13). In a normal wet swallow, these two contractile segments form a diagonal pressure band, corresponding to the peristaltic wave traversing the entire length of the esophagus. The contraction slope decreases as the peristalsis reaches the phrenic ampulla of the esophagus, and bolus front velocity decreases before it enters the stomach.

Peristalsis

The main function of the esophagus is to deliver a food bolus from the oral cavity to the stomach. The normal transfer of the food bolus requires coordinated, sequential contraction along the length of the esophagus. Normal esophageal contractions are called *primary peristalsis*. On esophageal manometry, the primary peristalsis is seen as a diagonal pressure band, as demonstrated in Figure 2.1, preceded by the UES opening with the onset of a wet swallow.

Secondary peristalsis occurs as a "housekeeping" reflex. As seen in Figure 2.14, when the primary peristalsis fails, this secondary peristalsis is initiated in the proximal esophagus without preceding UES relaxation (i.e., without swallow). In normal

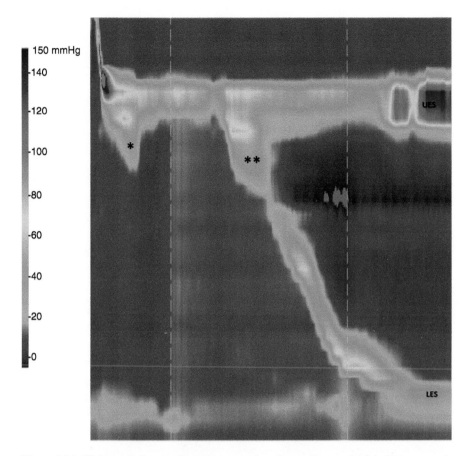

Figure 2.14 High-resolution esophageal manometry of secondary peristalsis. This wet swallow does not lead to a primary esophageal peristalsis in the smooth muscle esophagus. The onset of the peristaltic contractions in the striated esophagus is intact (*asterisk*), but there is a subsequent secondary peristalsis that is not immediately preceded by UES relaxation (*double asterisks*). The UES remains closed, with persistent higher pressure (*red hues*). This is a "housekeeping" mechanism to clear the esophagus of any residual bolus

subjects, it does generate a diagonal pressure band traversing the entire esophageal length. Tertiary waves, simultaneous contractions that are non-peristaltic, can happen in normal subjects as well as those with esophageal dysmotility. In isolation, the significance of tertiary waves is not known (Fig. 2.15).

Respiratory Variations in the Body of the Esophagus

As discussed earlier for landmark identification of PIP, the body of the esophagus is in the thoracic cavity. Therefore, the pressure variation seen on high-resolution esophageal manometry reflects the pressure pattern in the thoracic

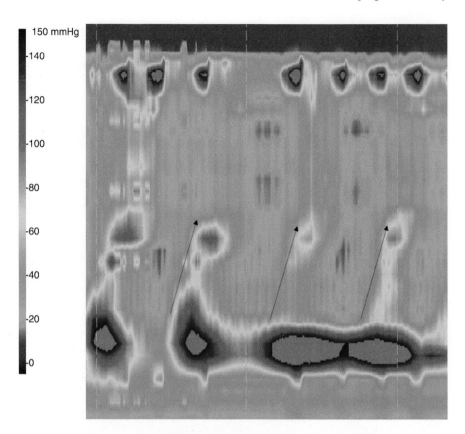

Figure 2.15 High-resolution esophageal manometry of tertiary contraction. Tertiary contractions are abnormal, retrograde contractions seen in the distal esophagus (*black arrows*). The LES appears to be hypertensive. These esophageal contractions may be seen in subjects with achalasia type III

cavity (Fig. 2.16). With inspiration, the pressure becomes negative, appearing dark blue on the pressure color plot. During expiration, the thoracic cavity pressure becomes positive, appearing as a hotter color. During inspiration, diaphragmatic crural contraction is easily noticeable.

Normal Bolus Pressure

Normal bolus pressure, generated by the bolus transfer through the esophagus, is less than 30 mm Hg, which can be outlined by setting the isobaric pressure at a minimum of 30 mm Hg. Any increase in intrabolus pressure beyond 30 mm Hg is considered abnormal. Higher intrabolus pressure could be the result of compartmentalization with esophagogastric junction outflow obstruction, when the bolus is propelled antegrade against a non-relaxing LES; panesophageal pressurization in

Figure 2.16 High-resolution resting esophageal manometry of respiratory pressure variation in the thoracic esophagus. During inspiration (I), the intrathoracic pressure drops, as seen by cooler color on pressure topography; with expiration (E), the pressure rises. The inspiration also coincides with CD contraction. The respiratory variability in the morphology of the distal esophageal high-pressure zone, composed of the LES and the CD, is evident

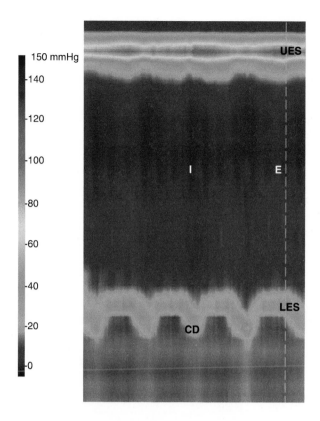

achalasia type II; or mixed contractions (premature and panesophageal pressurization) in achalasia type III. These patterns are discussed in detail later.

Gastric Pressure

Normal gastric pressure is approximately 10 mm Hg. During study analysis of esophageal manometry, the gastric pressure is set up in an area of no contraction, distal to the LES, as demonstrated in Figure 2.6. The LES pressure is calculated in relation to the gastric pressure. Therefore, the true basal LES pressure may be falsely underestimated if the gastric pressure is falsely elevated, as it may be in a person with abdominal obesity, for example.

Chicago Classification Parameters

The Chicago Classification of esophageal motility disorders, version 3.0 [1], uses a number of parameters for the interpretation of HRM recordings.

Integrated Relaxation Pressure (IRP)

With the onset of wet swallow and opening of the UES, the LES relaxes as well. Integrated relaxation pressure (IRP) is measured by the software as the mean of the 4 seconds of maximal deglutitive relaxation in the 10-second window from the onset of UES relaxation. The contributing times can be contiguous or non-contiguous (e.g., with the latter due to diaphragmatic contraction during inspiration). Normal IRP may vary depending on the manometry system used, but 15 mm Hg is considered the upper limit of normal with most software (Fig. 2.17).

There is a debate as to whether IRP should use the median (rather than the mean) of the 4 seconds of maximal deglutitive relaxation in the 10-second window. There is less likelihood that one or two outliers would impact the median, whereas they could greatly skew the mean result. The currently available software continues to take the mean of 4 seconds of maximal deglutitive relaxation in the 10-second window as the reported IRP, but a newer version using the median measurement will replace the mean.

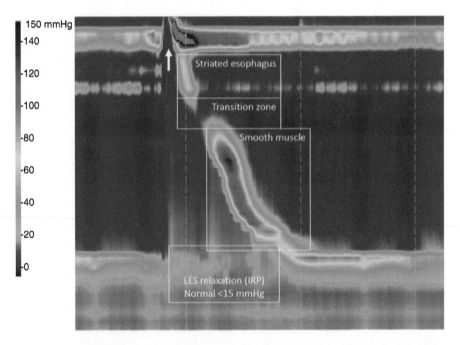

Figure 2.17 High-resolution manometry of normal Integrated relaxation pressure (IRP). With the onset of the wet swallow, the UES opens, followed by a normal primary peristalsis, depicted by the diagonal pressure band. The proximal striated esophagus is separated by the transition zone from the distal smooth muscle esophagus. The LES relaxes shortly after the UES opening with the onset of the wet swallow. The integrated relaxation pressure (IRP) is the mean of the 4 seconds of maximum deglutitive relaxation in a 10-second window from the onset of the UES relaxation

To measure IRP accurately, it is important to ensure that the 10-second window correctly outlines the true LES. The software may incorrectly recognize diaphragmatic contraction (such as in sliding hiatal hernia) as LES and therefore overestimates the IRP. With esophageal shortening, occasionally seen with achalasia or jackhammer esophagus, the LES is displaced proximally, which could spuriously lower LES relaxation pressure; therefore, the IRP should be carefully evaluated to ensure that it is not underestimated. Please refer to illustrations of achalasia with esophageal shortening for further detail.

Contractile Deceleration Point (CDP)

The contractile deceleration point (CDP) is an inflection point along the 30 mm Hg isobaric contour, at which the slope of the contraction decreases (Fig. 2.18). It represents the point where the bolus enters the phrenic ampulla on esophageal fluoroscopy. This globular structure is seen radiographically beneath the tubular esophagus

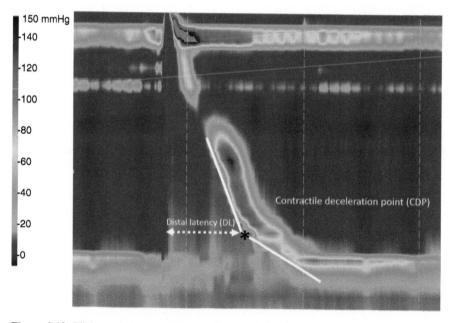

Figure 2.18 High-resolution manometry of normal Contractile deceleration point (CDP) and distal latency (DL). The solid white lines are tangential to the 30 mm Hg isobaric contours. The contractile deceleration point (CDP, *asterisk*) is the inflection point at which the tangent of the slope of the proximal solid line slows down, which corresponds to the point where the bolus at the end of the tubular esophagus reaches the phrenic ampulla. The distance (i.e., the time) between the onset of the UES relaxation and the CDP is referred to as distal latency (DL, *dotted line*). The normal DL is equal or greater than 4.5 seconds. A contraction with shortened DL is referred to as a *premature contraction*

and above the crural diaphragm (CD). It is essentially relaxed and effaced, elongating the LES, which empties between inspirations. The CDP is located within 3 cm of the LES. In circumstances where there is esophageal compartmentalization, the inflection point is along the isobaric contour line greater than the compartmentalized intrabolus pressure (*see* achalasia illustrations).

Distal Latency (DL)

Distal latency (DL), the interval on the x-axis between the UES opening and the CDP, is demonstrated in Figure 2.18. A normal DL is is equal or greater than 4.5 seconds. It is a measurement of deglutitive relaxation.

With the onset of the wet swallow, the vagus nerve initially activates the myenteric inhibitory neurons, releasing nitric oxide. This is followed by a delayed activation of the cholinergic pathway in the vagal fibers, once the sequential deglutitive inhibition has terminated. Moving distally along the esophagus, there is a gradual increase in the number of inhibitory noncholinergic (nitrergic) neurons and a decrease in the number of excitatory cholinergic neurons, resulting in the gradual increase in duration of deglutitive inhibition and a coordinated peristaltic wave. In individuals with distal esophageal spasm (*see* Fig. 2.39), deglutitive inhibition is reduced or absent, leading to a premature contraction and therefore a lower distal latency.

Distal Contractile Integral (DCI)

Distal contractile integral (DCI) is the contraction vigor exceeding 20 mm Hg isobaric contour in the distal two thirds of the esophagus, between the transition zone and the proximal margin of the LES. It is a composite measure of pressure amplitude, duration, and length of contraction (mmHg.sec.cm) (Fig. 2.19). A normal contraction has a minimum DCI of 450 mmHg.sec.cm to a maximum of 8000 mmHg. sec.cm. Any contraction with DCI of 100–450 mmHg.sec.cm is considered "weak," and any contraction with DCI less than 100 mmHg.sec.cm is categorized as "a failed swallow." If a contraction has DCI greater than 8000 mmHg.sec.cm, it is considered "hypercontractile." A "hypertensive" designation for contractions with DCI between 5000 and 8000 mmHg.sec.cm has no apparent clinical significance, so it is no longer reported in high-resolution esophageal manometry.

Contraction Patterns

As discussed above, a normal contraction pattern on esophageal manometry consists of a peristaltic contraction that is seen as a diagonal band started from the UES and extending to the LES, with the transition zone separating the striated esophagus

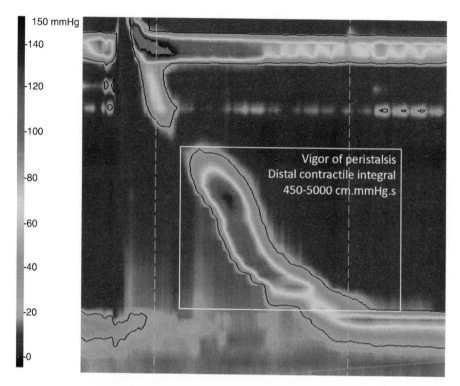

Figure 2.19 High-resolution esophageal manometry of normal Distal contractile integral (DCI). Based on the Chicago Classification V3.0., the contraction vigor of the second and third esophageal contractile segments (in the rectangle) is measured by the distal contractile integral (DCI), a composite value of pressure amplitude, duration, and length of the contraction

from the area of smooth muscle contraction. A "failed" swallow (DCI <100 mmHg. sec.cm) and a "weak" contraction (DCI 100–450 mmHg.sec.cm) are considered *ineffective*, but they are still considered peristaltic as long as they have a discernable diagonal shape (Figs. 2.20 and 2.21). There is not 100% agreement about these cut-off values, so values close to these cut-offs should be interpreted in conjunction with clinical data and impedance results, if available.

Any contraction with DL less than 4.5 seconds and normal contractile vigor (DCI >450 mmHg.sec.cm) is considered *premature* (Fig. 2.22). A weak contraction with DCI <450 mmHg.sec.cm with a reduced DL is considered "failed."

A peristaltic wave with DCI >8000 mmHg.sec.cm is considered *hypercontractile* (Fig. 2.23).

A *fragmented* contraction is demonstrated by a large break (>5 cm) in the 20 mm Hg isobaric contour with normal DCI (Fig. 2.24). If both a large break and a weak contraction coexist, the ineffective swallow (reported as DCI <450 mmHg.sec.cm) takes precedence over the fragmented contraction. Fragmented contractions have been found to be more common in patients with dysphagia than in control subjects [2, 3]. Small breaks (2–5 cm in length) are of unclear significance and occur occasionally in normal subjects, so they are no longer required to be reported.

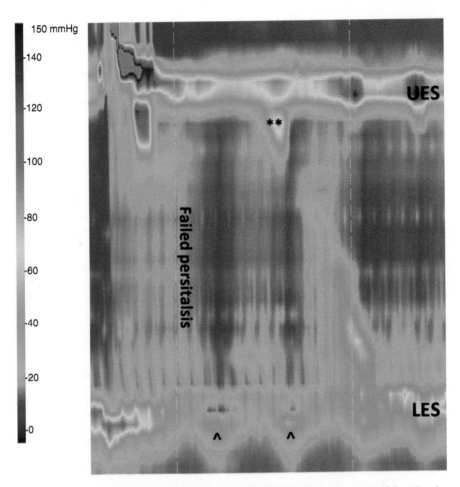

Figure 2.20 High-resolution esophageal manometry of failed primary peristalsis. After the onset of the wet swallow, marked by normal relaxation of the UES, the proximal striated esophagus contracts, but the peristalsis does not propagate beyond the striated esophagus. A secondary peristalsis (*double asterisks*) is triggered 5 seconds later and results in propagating contraction along the length of the esophagus. Note that there is no preceding UES relaxation before the secondary peristalsis. CD contraction with inspiration (*arrowheads*) is also seen

Pressurization Patterns

The normal intrabolus pressure is less than 30 mm Hg, which is essentially the pressure generated by esophageal peristalsis. Therefore, intrabolus pressure patterns are defined using the 30 mm Hg isobaric contour. Abnormal pressurization corresponds to regions of esophageal pressurization greater than 30 mm Hg. With "panesophageal pressurization," there is a column of pressure spanning from the UES to the

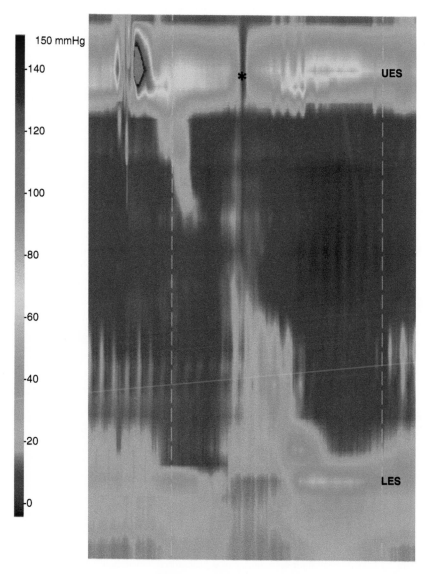

Figure 2.21 High-resolution esophageal manometry of a weak peristalsis. The DCI is found to be less than 450 mmHg.sec.cm. The *asterisk* indicates a belch, marked by a brief interruption in the UES resting pressure

EGJ. "Compartmentalized" pressurization is seen when the pressure column extends from the deglutitive contractile front to the EGJ. This compartmentalized pressurization could represent bolus retention in the esophagus, which is better seen with impedance. In the setting of hiatal hernia, pressurization may be restricted to the zone between the LES and CD, which is referred to as "EGJ pressurization."

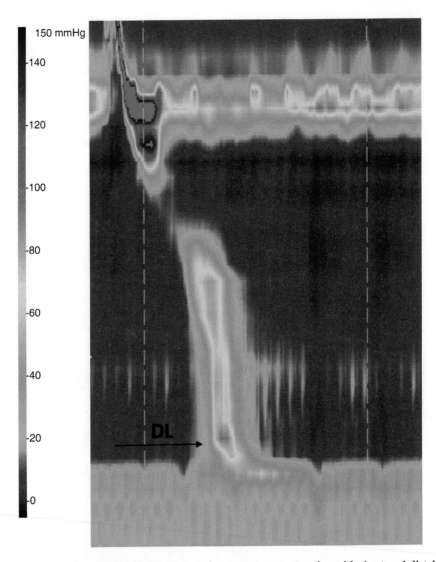

Figure 2.22 High-resolution manometry of a premature contraction with shortened distal latency. The HRM plot shows normal UES relaxation, and there is a peristaltic contraction with normal contraction vigor, but it appears premature, with shortened DL of 3.8 seconds (normal ≥4.5 sec). The presence of a peristaltic wave and the LES relaxation rule out achalasia type III (spastic). As per Chicago Classification V3.0, at least two premature contractions are required to diagnose distal esophageal spasm (DES). This esophageal dysmotility is thought to be due to inadequate deglutitive inhibition, with loss of non-cholinergic neurons in the distal esophagus

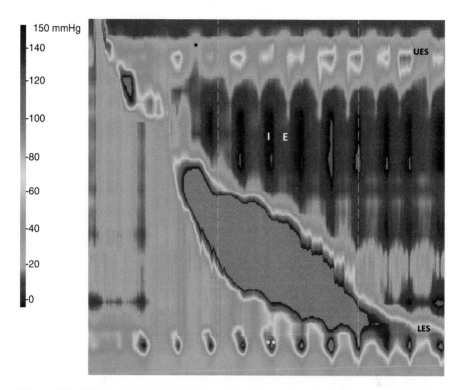

Figure 2.23 High-resolution esophageal manometry of a hypercontractile swallow. The esophageal peristalsis pressure is significantly elevated; the contraction vigor (DCI) is measured at 19,220 mmHg.sec.cm. This significantly hypercontractile esophageal contraction may cause transient chest pain and dysphagia. The integrated relaxation pressure (IRP) is normal, at 10.4 mm Hg. As per the Chicago Classification V3.0, at least two hypercontractile wet swallows with DCI greater than 8000 mm Hg are required to diagnose jackhammer esophagus. The *asterisk* shows belching, as demonstrated by a transient relaxation of the UES. CD contraction (*double asterisks*) is in phase with lower intrathoracic pressure during inspiration (I)

Contractile Front Velocity (CFV)

To measure contractile front velocity (CFV), the isobaric contour is set at 30 mm Hg. The slope of the tangential line along this isobaric contour between the proximal smooth muscle esophageal contraction and the CDP is known as CFV. The normal value of CFV is less than 9 cm/sec. The significance of CFV is unknown. In the past, any contraction with CFV greater than 9 cm/sec was labelled as "rapid contraction," but this parameter has now fallen out of favor; the most recent Chicago Classification does not require it for the diagnosis of any abnormalities.

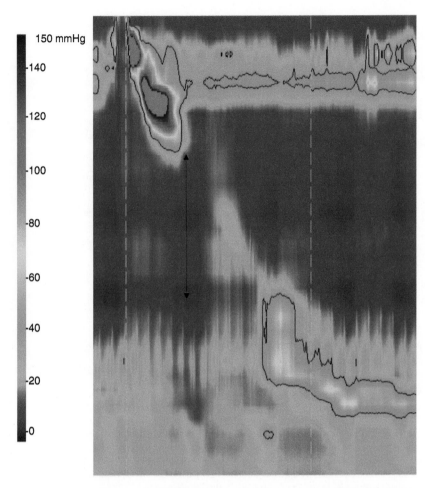

Figure 2.24 High-resolution esophageal manometry of fragmented peristalsis. In this example, the UES opens normally with the onset of the wet swallow and the striated esophageal contraction is normal, but there is a 9-cm break in the 20 mm Hg isobaric contour (*arrow*) consistent with a large break (i.e. greater than 5 cm). The contraction vigor (DCI) is 458 mmHg.sec.cm. According to the Chicago Classification V3.0, to meet the criteria for *fragmented peristalsis* (known as a minor esophageal motility disorder), at least 50% of wet swallows must have large breaks with normal DCI (450–8000 mmHg.sec.cm)

Classification of Esophageal Motility Disorders

The most updated Chicago Classification, version 3.0 [1], utilizes a hierarchical approach to primarily recognize major esophageal motility disorders as patterns of motor dysfunction that are not encountered in normal subjects with normal EGJ relaxation. These conditions are subdivided further to disorders of EGJ outflow (achalasia subtypes I to III and EGJ outflow obstruction) and major disorders of peristalsis (absent contractility, distal esophageal spasm, and jackhammer esophagus). On the other hand, the clinical significance of minor motility disorders, including ineffective esophageal motility and fragmented peristalsis, characterized by impaired bolus transit, continue to be actively debated [4]; however, they are thought to be associated with impaired bolus clearance. The following sections further discuss individual disorders.

Achalasia

Achalasia is an esophageal motility disorder resulting from inflammation and progressive degeneration of ganglion cells in the myenteric plexus. The inflammatory process predominantly affects nitric oxide–producing inhibitory neurons and affects esophageal smooth muscle relaxation, whereas the cholinergic neurons that contribute to LES tone may be relatively spared. The imbalance between cholinergic and nitric oxide–producing neurons impairs peristaltic contraction in the smooth muscle esophagus and impairs the LES relaxation.

Interestingly, opioid use has also been shown to mimic manometric findings of esophagogastric junction outflow obstruction and achalasia by creating a hypertensive LES and incomplete relaxation of the LES, particularly type III achalasia. Therefore, it is important to review the patient's medication history [4].

Subjects with achalasia often present with dysphagia, regurgitation, chest pain, heartburn, and sometimes weight loss. On barium esophagogram, the classic appearance of "bird-beak," caused by a tight LES, can be seen. In some cases, aperistaltic, dilated esophagus with delayed esophageal barium emptying is also appreciated. On upper endoscopy, the body of the esophagus may elicit abnormal contractions, and the LES may be perceived to be tight, with lack of relaxation on air insufflation or even difficulty in traversing the esophagus during the upper endoscopy. In severe cases, the esophageal lumen may be dilated, with cobblestoning appearance, and residual food debris may be seen, with stasis esophagitis. Upper endoscopy has low sensitivity for the accurate diagnosis of achalasia. Therefore, esophageal manometry is crucial to differentiate achalasia from other esophagogastric junction outflow obstructions.

Achalasia is subdivided into three types: *Type I* (*classic achalasia*) is diagnosed when there is lack of LES relaxation, demonstrated by 100% failed peristalsis, elevated mean IRP (on the Medtronic® system, >15 mm Hg), and DCI less than 100 mHg.sec.cm (Figs. 2.25 and 2.26). Any premature, weak contraction with DCI <450 mmHg.sec.cm and DL less than 4.5 seconds also satisfies the criteria for failed peristalsis. Note that the normal IRP cut-off may vary on different manometric systems. In some systems, the upper limit of normal IRP may be as low as 10 mm Hg, so if the IRP is borderline, the diagnosis of achalasia should always be entertained in patients with aperistalsis.

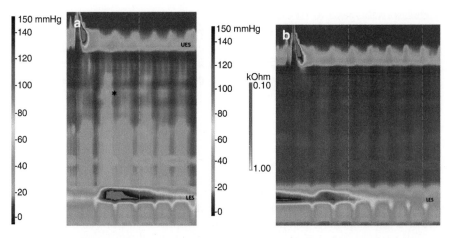

Figure 2.25 High-resolution esophageal manometry of achalasia type I. A, One wet swallow is shown, which leads to appropriate opening of the UES. There is no peristaltic contraction along the length of the esophagus, as expected in achalasia. The proximal striated esophagus is not affected by achalasia, but in this figure the striated esophageal contraction is not present (*asterisk*). The LES does not relax in response to the wet swallow. The absence of peristaltic contraction and the lack of LES relaxation in response to wet swallows are the characteristic features of achalasia type I. **B,** High-resolution esophageal manometry with impedance in achalasia type I. Because of the lack of LES relaxation in response to wet swallows, bolus accumulation occurs in the esophagus, as seen by the column of low impedance (*purple*). The fluid level approaches the proximal esophagus, which can increase the risk of aspiration. Therefore, during the data acquisition, caution should be exercised in patients suspected to have achalasia, to minimize the risk of aspiration with subsequent swallows

Type II achalasia also has elevated mean IRP and 100% failed peristalsis, but in 10 wet swallows, at least two show panesophageal pressurization, seen as simultaneous isobaric pressure spanning the entire length of the esophagus (Figs. 2.27–2.30). The DCI should not be calculated, as contractions are not peristaltic. In addition, the esophagus may be shortened during panesophageal pressurization, which could make the IRP falsely normal. Proximal displacement of the LES should lend a clue, and cautious interpretation of IRP values should be implemented to avoid misdiagnosing achalasia.

Type III achalasia (spastic achalasia) is characterized by elevated mean IRP (>15 mm Hg) with no normal peristalsis but the presence of premature contractions, defined as distal latency less than 4.5 seconds, with normal DCI (>450 mmHg.sec. cm) (Figs. 2.31–2.34). Type III achalasia may also be mixed with panesophageal pressurization.

Figure 2.35 is an additional example of achalasia type III in a patient who has undergone a therapeutic intervention, a failed Heller's myotomy.

In patients with achalasia (particularly those with more advanced age), it is important to rule out other conditions that may mimic achalasia, such as intraluminal or extraluminal pathology at the distal esophagus, which may cause EGJ outflow obstruction. Figure 2.36 shows an example of pseudoachalasia.

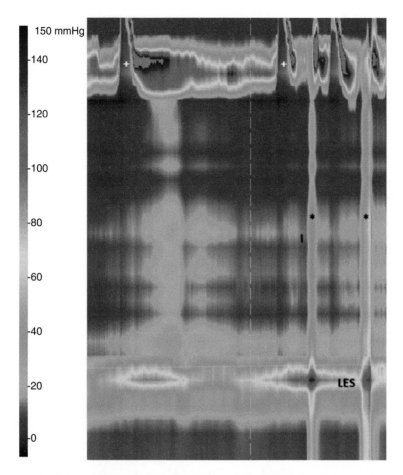

Figure 2.26 High-resolution esophageal manometry of achalasia type I. Two wet swallows (*plus signs*) are shown, as marked by the relaxation of the UES. However, there is no peristalsis throughout the esophagus. The LES does not relax, as evident by persistently high IRP. The absence of peristalsis and lack of LES relaxation with wet swallows are classic manometric findings of achalasia type I. A high-pressure column in the esophagus and the proximal stomach preceded by a deep inspiration (I) is due to a cough (*asterisk*). Dry heaving could generate the same manometric pattern, although it does not have the preceding negative pressure due to inspiration. These patterns associated with cough and dry heaving should not be confused with a panesophageal contraction

Generally, the bolus clearance is impaired in all subtypes of achalasia. During the data acquisition, the HRM operator should remain vigilant for fluid column accumulation and should advise the patient to report any symptoms, including chest pain, dysphagia, or fullness, as the latter could increase the risk of aspiration. Therefore, it may be prudent to turn on impedance during the data acquisition to actively assess bolus clearance.

Figure 2.27 High-resolution esophageal manometry of achalasia type II with esophageal shortening. Panesophageal pressurization leads to cephalic pull on the distal esophagus (*arrow*). The transient shortening of the esophagus may spuriously lower the IRP, but the LES IRP remains elevated at 37 mm Hg, which is greater than the normal 15 mm Hg. This is seen as no change in pressure color along the LES (*asterisk*). It remains significantly above the gastric pressure. Note the residual UES relaxation pressure, which is also increased (*double asterisks*). This pressure approximates the proximal esophageal pressure, so this rise in pressure is due to the panesophageal pressurization rather than to UES dysfunction

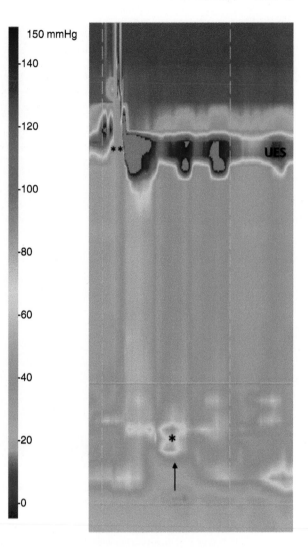

Esophagogastric Junction Outflow Obstruction (EGJOO)

Patients with esophagogastric junction outflow obstruction (EGJOO) present with various symptoms, including dysphagia, heartburn, regurgitation, retrosternal chest pain, and atypical symptoms of gastroesophageal reflux disease (GERD). Manometrically, EGJOO is characterized by incomplete LES relaxation, with elevated mean IRP greater than 15 mm Hg, but it does not meet criteria for achalasia (types I to III), as there is evidence of intact or weak peristalsis (Fig. 2.37). Nonetheless, some cases of EGJOO could progress to achalasia over time or may be the result of incompletely expressed achalasia.

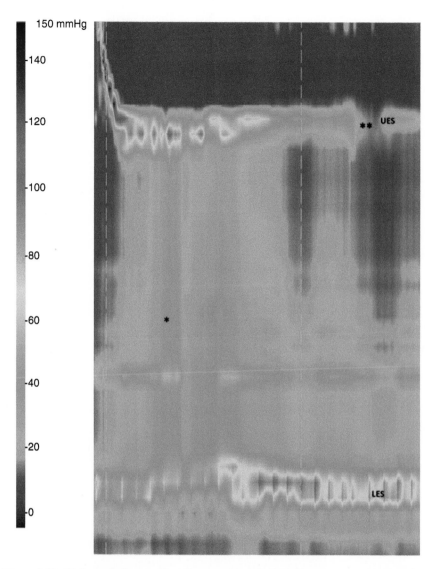

Figure 2.28 High-resolution esophageal manometry of achalasia type II with an esophageal vent. Here, a wet swallow leads to simultaneous isobaric pressure spanning the entire length of the esophagus, referred to as "panesophageal pressurization" (*asterisk*). The LES does not relax. In achalasia patients, transient UES opening (*double asterisks*), an esophageal vent, serves as a relieving mechanism that may or may not be associated with concomitant LES relaxation, which could allow the intra-esophageal content to enter the stomach and further relieve the esophageal pressure. There is also a secondary wave of panesophageal pressurization

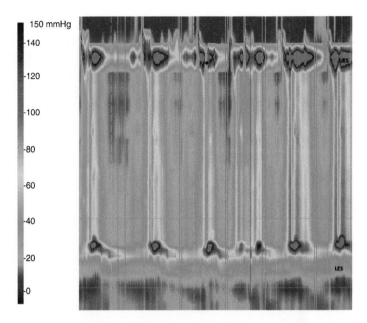

Figure 2.29 High-resolution esophageal manometry of achalasia type II. Shown are multiple swallows with the classic finding of panesophageal pressurization and subtle cephalic displacement of the LES during the pressurization. There is no peristaltic contraction, and the LES relaxation pressure has increased. This HRM is highly characteristic of achalasia type II

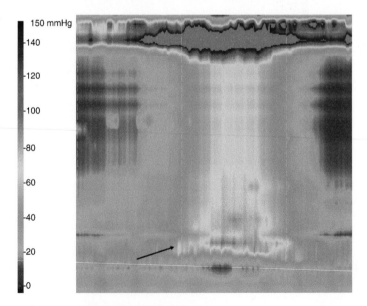

Figure 2.30 High-resolution esophageal manometry of a massive secondary contraction with panesophageal pressurization in a subject with known type II achalasia. Because of significant pressurization along the entire length of the esophagus, the LES is pulled slightly cephalically, resulting in esophageal shortening (*arrow*). Note that the UES pressure is also transiently increased during the secondary contraction. This phenomenon occurs with the contraction of the longitudinal muscles without engagement of the circular muscles

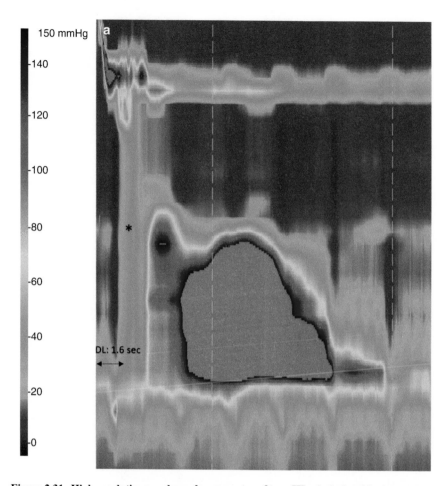

Figure 2.31 High-resolution esophageal manometry of type III achalasia with vigorous contraction. A, In this HRM, the UES opens appropriately in response to a wet swallow, but it does not lead to a peristaltic contraction. Instead, it produces a vigorous contraction, as demonstrated by shortened distal latency (DL) of 1.6 seconds. (Normal DL is ≥4.5 seconds.) The vigorous contraction is preceded by a transient panesophageal compartmentalization (*asterisk*). This should not be confused with type II achalasia, given the subsequent vigorous contraction. The LES does not relax, as evident from the IRP of 30 mm Hg (normal <15 mm Hg). **B,** The impedance is shown in purple and demonstrates the presence of fluid bolus. The UES opens with the onset of the wet swallow. There is proximal esophageal bolus escape (*asterisk*), but the bolus lingers in the distal half of the esophagus because of incomplete LES relaxation. Ultimately, it does not clear completely at the end of the vigorous contraction

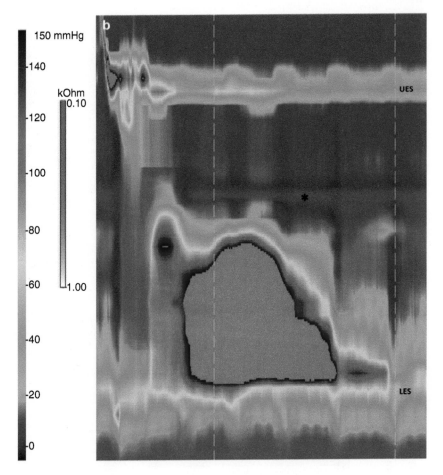

Figure 2.31 (continued)

   Given the outflow obstruction, a mechanical obstruction at the gastroesophageal junction (such as a stricture, esophageal wall stiffness due to infiltrative diseases, or malignancy) should be ruled out. Upper endoscopy, endoscopic ultrasound, and cross-sectional imaging, if clinically indicated, should be considered. Other possible causes include vascular obstruction of the distal esophagus or a large sliding or para-esophageal hiatal hernia. Figure 2.38 demonstrates the manometric findings in a patient with EGJOO who underwent laparoscopic insertion of a LINX® magnetic LES sphincter augmentation device for refractory GERD with hiatal hernia.

Distal Esophageal Spasm (DES)

The underlying pathophysiology of distal esophageal spasm (DES) is unknown. It is associated with an impairment of deglutitive inhibitory innervation, leading to premature and rapid contractions in the distal esophagus, which may be due to dysfunction

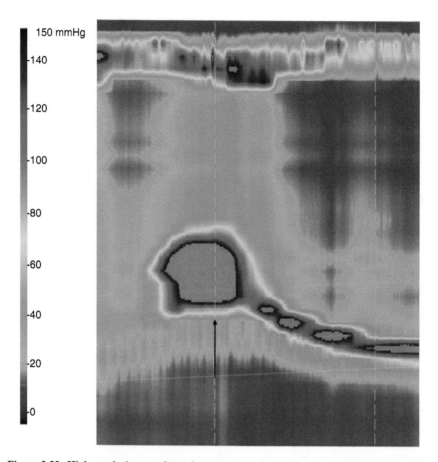

Figure 2.32 High-resolution esophageal manometry of spontaneous esophageal shortening in achalasia type III. This is another HRM finding in the same patient as Figure 2.31 with achalasia type III. In this HRM, the isolated contraction is not preceded by a wet swallow, as there is no relaxation in the UES, therefore, this is a secondary contraction. Note the esophageal pressurization and esophageal shortening, as seen by the cephalic displacement of the LES (*arrow*)

and/or degradation of nitric oxide–producing neurons. Patients may present with dysphagia and retrosternal chest pain; some may report heartburn or regurgitation.

Manometrically, DES is diagnosed when the patient has a normal mean IRP and normal DCI (>450 mmHg.sec.cm) but a shortened DL (<4.5 seconds) in 20% or more of wet swallows (Fig. 2.39; *see also* Fig. 2.22). It is not uncommon to see some normal peristalsis.

Jackhammer Esophagus (Hypercontractile Esophagus)

In contrast to DES, in which the primary pathology is thought to be dysfunction of inhibitory neurons, jackhammer esophagus is thought to be due to overactivity of excitatory innervation, or smooth-muscle response to excitatory neurons. Clinical

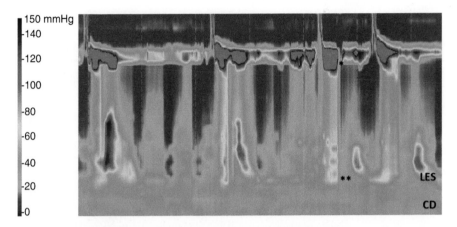

Figure 2.33 High-resolution esophageal manometry of four wet swallows in achalasia type III with esophageal vent. These esophageal contractions are vigorous and premature, with distal latency of 1.8 seconds. The IRP of the LES is 22 mm Hg, compared with a normal IRP of ≤15 mm Hg. Therefore, the study meets the criteria for achalasia type III. Subjects with achalasia tend to have esophageal venting to decrease the intra-esophageal pressure by relaxation of the UES (*asterisk*), which may transiently relax the LES (*double asterisks*). Note that there is also a sliding hiatal hernia, as evident from the separation between the LES and CD

symptoms include retrosternal chest pain, dysphagia, and occasionally GERD that is resistant to treatment with proton pump inhibitors (PPIs).

On high-resolution esophageal manometry, patients are required to have at least two swallows with DCI greater than 8000 mmHg.sec.cm (Fig. 2.40). Because of its significant overlap with control subjects, "nutcracker esophagus" or "hypertensive peristalsis" with DCI greater than 5000 mmHg.sec.cm is no longer reported as a disorder of peristalsis.

Absent Contractility (Aperistalsis)

On esophageal manometry, patients with aperistalsis have no scorable contractions in 100% of swallows (Fig. 2.41). Congruently, multiple rapid swallows do not lead to a peristaltic wave in this condition. A workup of these patients should be considered to look for underlying autoimmune rheumatologic diseases such as systemic sclerosis, Sjögren's syndrome, systemic lupus erythematosus, polymyositis, dermatomyositis, mixed connective tissue disease, or paraneoplastic syndrome (e.g., anti-Hu antibodies in small cell lung cancer). About 20% of patients with absent contractility do not have rheumatologic diseases; other causes can include severe GERD, chronic radiation esophagitis, autonomic and peripheral neuropathies, and neurodegenerative diseases such as multiple sclerosis. In addition, incompletely expressed achalasia may be suspected, especially with borderline elevated mean IRP.

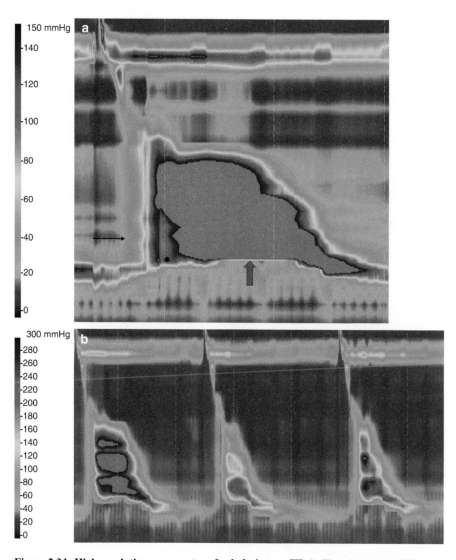

Figure 2.34 High-resolution manometry of achalasia type III. A, There is normal UES relaxation but no peristaltic contraction in the body of the esophagus. The contraction is premature, with a shortened DL of 2.3 seconds (*thin arrow*). The LES relaxation pressure is increased (*asterisk*), with IRP of 20 mm Hg. Note that there is esophageal shortening due to spastic contraction, and the distal esophagus is pulled upward (*thick arrow*). Given the absence of peristaltic contractions and shortened DL, this HRM is diagnostic of achalasia type III, rather than EGJ outflow obstruction (which has normal peristalsis) or distal esophageal spasm (which has normal peristaltic contraction and normal IRP). **B,** In the same patient, when the maximum pressure range is increased to 300 mm Hg, a peculiar reproducible pattern is observed. "Stacks of sandbags" correspond to esophageal diverticula, which can be seen with endoscopy (**C**) and barium esophagogram (**D**). There are large and small diverticula in the body of the esophagus, likely due to longstanding spastic contraction, esophageal dysmotility, and lack of LES relaxation. The LES is quite tightly pinched, owing to achalasia, despite air insufflation on the upper endoscopy. This is more noticeable with the "bird-beak" appearance on the barium esophagogram

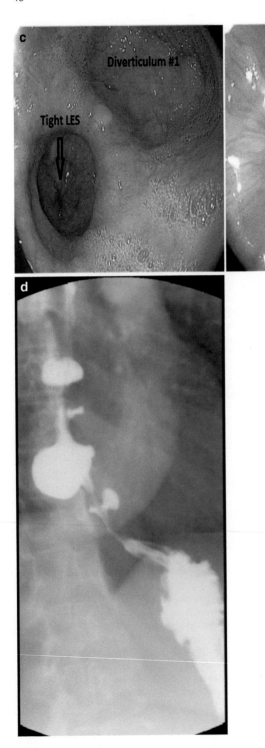

Figure 2.34 (continued)

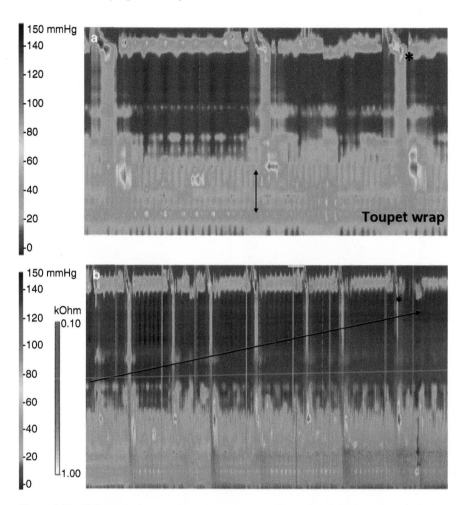

Figure 2.35 High-resolution esophageal manometry after a failed Heller's myotomy with Toupet fundoplication in a patient with achalasia type III. A, The patient had ongoing dysphagia. The surgical myotomy is only 4 cm in length (*arrow*), which is not enough, given the persistent HRM finding of spastic contraction of the smooth muscle above the myotomized esophagus (i.e., intrathoracic esophagus). The horizontal band of high pressure corresponds to the Toupet wrap. The wrap is relatively tight. Patients with achalasia often belch shortly after the swallow (*asterisk*) to vent the esophagus and lower the built-up intraesophageal pressure. Patients often respond to a longer, intra-thoracic esophageal myotomy and revision of the Toupet wrap. **B,** High-resolution esophageal manometry with impedance in the same patient. As the LES does not relax appropriately, the fluid bolus gradually builds up in the esophagus over multiple wet swallows, which is easily appreciated on the impedance. The *arrow* shows the gradual accumulation of the column of fluid. This finding is similar to a timed-barium esophagogram

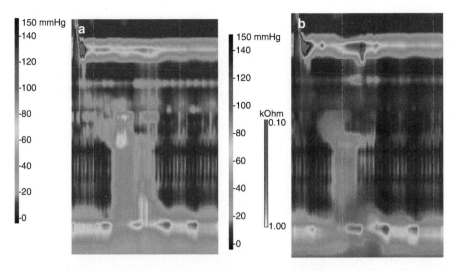

Figure 2.36 High-resolution esophageal manometry of pseudoachalasia. A, The UES opens normally in response to a wet swallow, but there is no normal primary esophageal peristalsis along the length of the esophagus. There is a subsequent esophageal compartmentalization, as seen by a vertical high-pressure column. The IRP is 37 mm Hg, consistent with abnormal LES relaxation. The manometric study is concerning for achalasia type III, but it is prudent to have endoscopic evaluation and cross-sectional imaging (if clinically warranted), to rule out obstructive distal esophageal pathologies, including stricture, webs, malignancy (both intraluminal or extraluminal tumors), or infiltrative diseases. This patient was found to have hepatocellular carcinoma metasta-sizing to the distal esophagus, seen on cross-sectional imaging with a normal upper endoscopy. **B,** Impedance in pseudoachalasia showed a bolus escape in the proximal esophagus. Again, the LES does not relax after the onset of the wet swallow, so there is the bolus holdup in the distal esopha-gus and the bolus does not clear completely, as demonstrated by persistent lower impedance (*purple*) at the end of the wet swallow

Figure 2.37 High-resolution esophageal manometry of esophagogastric junction outflow obstruction (EGJOO). A, Peristaltic contraction is seen in the body of the esophagus, and the UES opens appropriately with the onset of wet swallows. The LES remains contracted, however, as depicted by a high-pressure zone. The IRP in this case is 21 mm Hg, greater than the normal IRP of ≤15 mm Hg. This HRM finding may be seen with large hiatal hernias or an infiltrative esopha-geal disorder (e.g., amyloidosis, esophageal wall tumors, linitis plastica of the esophagus). It may also evolve into achalasia once the peristalsis is lost. Generally, cross-sectional imaging of the distal esophagus with CT scan or endoscopic ultrasound is warranted to rule out these diagnoses. **B,** Lower impedance is seen, with salt-water bolus present in the esophagus. There is a "shelving" effect in the distal esophagus (*dotted line*), where the bolus is held up for 2.7 seconds. This effect is due to the inadequate LES relaxation. The pressure build-up in the distal esophagus acts as a "piston" and ultimately overcomes the LES pressure; subsequently, the bolus clears the distal esophagus. This HRM finding is nonspecific and could also occur with deep inspiration causing diaphragmatic contraction, or a transient increase in the high-pressure zone composed of the LES and CD. In this HRM, the bolus ultimately clears the esophagus completely

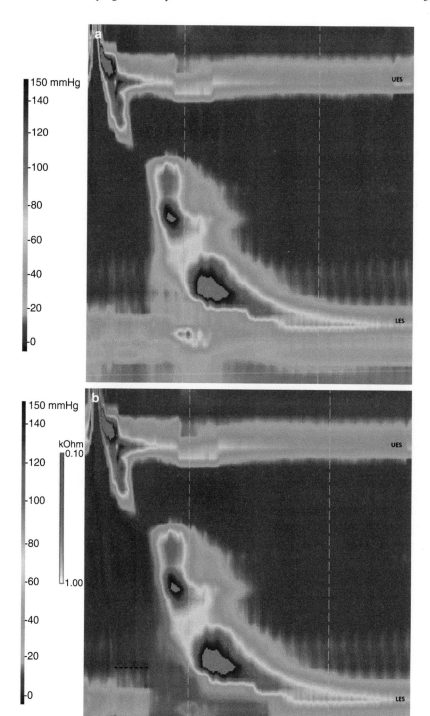

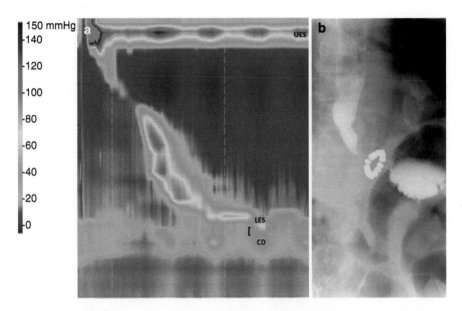

Figure 2.38 High-resolution esophageal manometry of a sliding hiatal hernia (LINX® insertion). A, On esophageal manometry before insertion of the LINX® device, the UES opens normally in response to the onset of the wet swallow. Shortly after, the LES relaxes. A second horizontal pressure band fluctuates in conjunction with the respiratory cycles, consistent with contraction of the CD. The pressure inversion point is along the CD. There is a small hiatal hernia (*bracket*), measuring 2–3 cm in size. **B,** A barium esophagogram of the same patient shows the LINX® device in situ. The device was inserted for refractory GERD after a positive Bravo™ pH study showed an increased number of symptomatic refluxes. This image shows a "bird-beak" appearance suggestive of pseudoachalasia at the distal esophagus, but the barium does traverse the EGJ, with contrast ultimately appearing in the proximal stomach. **C,** After the LINX® procedure, the patient reported dysphagia and underwent esophageal HRM, which showed a normal peristaltic contraction with elevated (but still normal) contraction vigor (DCI <8000 mmHg.sec.cm). The IRP has increased from the normal IRP at baseline. This HRM is suggestive of EGJOO, likely due to the LINX® device, a finding that corresponds well to the barium finding. **D,** After removal of the LINX® device and adhesionolysis, the patient's symptoms resolved. HRM shows normalization of the IRP, and the wet swallow leads to a normal peristaltic esophageal contraction

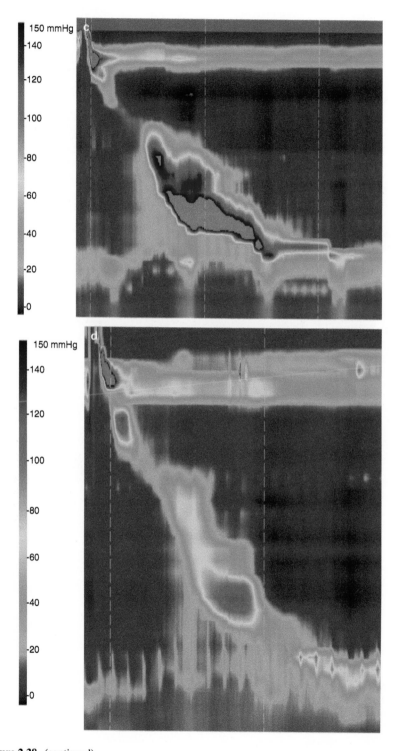

Figure 2.38 (continued)

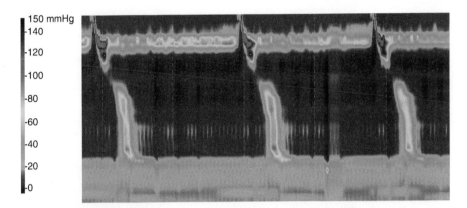

Figure 2.39 High-resolution esophageal manometry of multiple wet swallows in diffuse esophageal spasm (DES). These three peristaltic contractions occur prematurely, with distal latency (DL) of 3.5–3.8 seconds. (Normal is ≥4.5 seconds.) Because there are more than two swallows with premature contraction, this HRM is diagnostic for DES. The contraction vigor (DCI) is normal. The lower esophageal sphincter relaxes normally; the IRP is <15 mm Hg

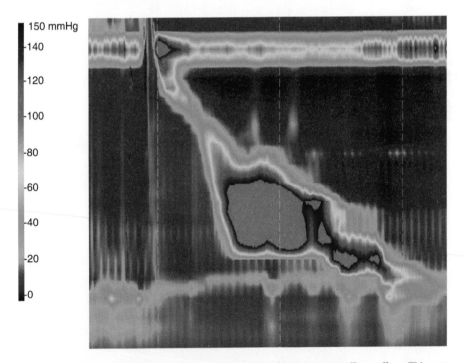

Figure 2.40 High-resolution esophageal manometry of hypercontractile swallow. This wet swallow shows normal peristaltic contraction, with normal IRP and DL, but the contraction vigor (DCI) is significantly increased, being greater than 8000 mmHg.sec.cm. Two or more of these hypercontractile swallows are required to diagnose *jackhammer esophagus*

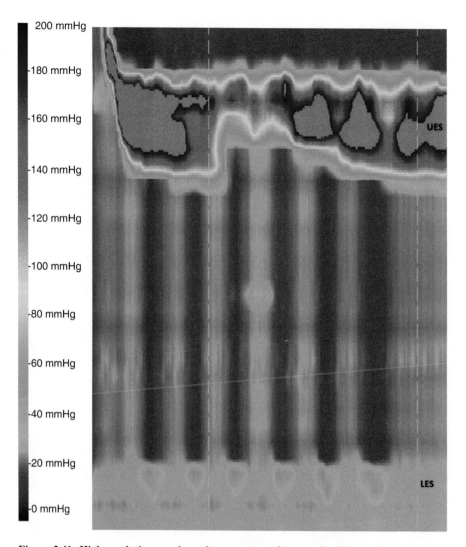

Figure 2.41 High-resolution esophageal manometry of an aperistaltic esophagus and low LES resting pressure. This type of HRM may be seen in patients with connective tissue disorders such as scleroderma. It is a common finding in absent contractility (major motility disorder) and occasionally can be seen in ineffective esophageal motility (minor motility disorder). Note that the proximal striated esophagus is intact, with peristaltic contractions. Interestingly, the UES resting pressure is elevated at 155 mm Hg, but it opens completely. This finding may be due to catheter irritation of the hypopharynx, resulting in a gagging sensation, compounded by the subject's anxiety during the study. Other differentials include cervical osteophytes. UES relaxation pressure is normal; therefore, cricopharyngeal bar is unlikely. The patient does have tachypnea, with a respiratory rate of 30/minute, which can represent anxiety or restrictive/obstructive lung disease. In the setting of aperistaltic esophagus, which can occur in association with connective tissue disease, interstitial lung disease should be investigated

Ineffective Esophageal Motility (IEM)

Ineffective esophageal motility (IEM) is defined as 50% or more of wet swallows considered failed or weak, with DCI less than 450 mmHg.sec.cm. As per the Chicago Classification V3.0, the unifying feature of swallows contributing to this diagnosis is poor bolus transit in the distal esophagus (Fig. 2.42). There is no need to make a distinction between failed swallows and weak swallows, eliminating the

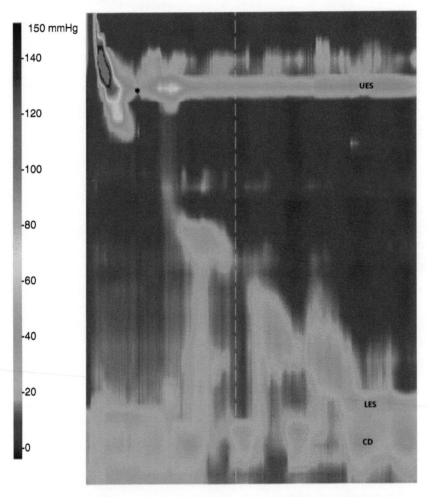

Figure 2.42 High-resolution esophageal manometry of ineffective esophageal motility (IEM). The UES relaxes in response to a wet swallow. The esophageal contraction is propagating with a peristaltic wave, but the contraction vigor (DCI) is 125 mmHg.sec.cm. Based on the Chicago Classification V3.0, this is considered a weak contraction. IEM is diagnosed when at least 50% of wet swallows have weak contractions. This is a minor esophageal dysmotility, which could be a primary esophageal motor disorder or could be secondary to GERD, eosinophilic esophagitis, scleroderma, or another connective tissue disorder. In this HRM, there is also a 2-cm sliding hiatal hernia, demonstrated by a separation between the LES and the (CD) contraction. The CD contracts with inspiration, as noted by respiratory cycling of pressure variation along the CD. There is also a small belch shortly after the swallow (*asterisk*), as demonstrated by transient UES opening

former designation of "frequent failed peristalsis," given the 83% positive agreement and 90% negative agreement in a validation sample of 100 patients [5]. This DCI level is not a hard cut-off, however, and the correlation between DCI and bolus transit is not perfect. Hence, manometric findings of IEM should be interpreted in conjunction with clinical data and, if available, impedance results. The presentation of patients with IEM can be heterogenous, and they may be asymptomatic. Common presentations of IEM are heartburn, dysphagia, regurgitation, and chest pain. Less common symptoms include chronic cough, hoarseness, sore throat, indigestion, belching, odynophagia, or choking. IEM can be associated with suboptimally controlled GERD; esophageal ring, webs, or stricture; eosinophilic, infectious, or radiation esophagitis; or side effects of medications.

Certain provocative tests may be considered in assessing subjects with IEM. One of these provocative tests is multiple rapid swallows (MRS), in which the patient is asked to take five swallows with 10 mL of water within 10 seconds (Fig. 2.43). The MRS provokes a deglutitive inhibition of the esophageal body, while LES tone is maintained until the last swallow. This method assesses esophageal peristaltic reserve and is particularly helpful in assessing IEM, as an intact MRS suggests intact neural and muscular functions. An appropriate response to MRS is seen when the ratio of the DCI generated by the peristaltic contraction at the end of MRS is greater than the mean DCI of the 10 wet swallows [6]. There are no optimal criteria for abnormal MRS in IEM. Other criteria have been evaluated to help identify IEM, such as the evidence of bolus retention on impedance, or the pattern of failed or weak swallows, or the degree of bolus retention seen with each swallow [2, 3], but these studies have not been able to consistently diagnose IEM, and it is important to note that IEM can be seen occasionally in asymptomatic patients.

Fragmented Peristalsis

Subjects with fragmented peristalsis have 50% or more fragmented contractions with DCI greater than 450 mmHg.sec.cm. Large breaks (>5 cm in length) in the 20 mm Hg isobaric contour are considered significant and should be counted for this diagnosis (Fig. 2.44). These patients may have dysphagia. Recent studies have shown that the large break in fragmented peristalsis may be associated with chronic cough [6], but it can also be seen in asymptomatic subjects.

High-Resolution Manometry Beyond the Chicago Classification

Cricopharyngeal Bar and Zenker's Diverticulum

Cricopharyngeal disorders contribute to dysphagia by impairing the bolus transit from the hypopharynx into the esophagus. Most patients describe symptoms suggestive of oropharyngeal dysphagia (Fig. 2.45). Videofluoroscopy of the pharynx

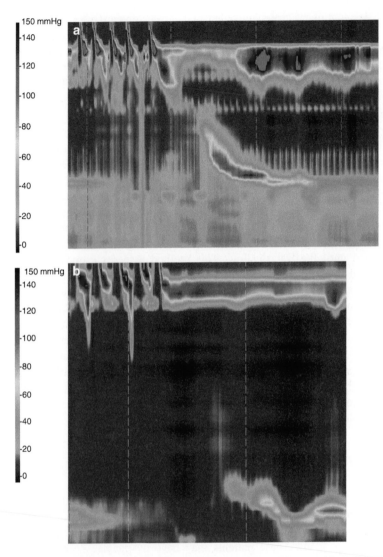

Figure 2.43 High-resolution esophageal manometry of "multiple rapid swallows" in a patient with IEM. Multiple rapid swallows (MRS) is a provocative test in which the subject takes five swallows of 5–10 mL of normal saline in rapid sequence, generally within 10 seconds. Normally, the MRS results in inhibition of peristalsis along the esophageal body and the LES. After the last swallow, normally there is a strong esophageal body peristaltic contraction and the LES regains its tone, a response referred to as *esophageal peristaltic reserve*. This response requires intact neuromuscular function. One study has shown that MRS has value in predicting esophageal transit symptoms such as dysphagia following anti-reflux surgery; these patients showed absent peristalsis after MRS. **A,** MRS led to a normal response with intact esophageal peristaltic reserve. The software can measure the DCI once the second and third contractile esophageal segments are highlighted. Note that this patient had a transient gag after the fourth swallow. **B,** In this MRS study of a different patient with IEM, no esophageal peristalsis is seen after the fifth wet swallow. The striated esophagus contracts, and the LES relaxes normally

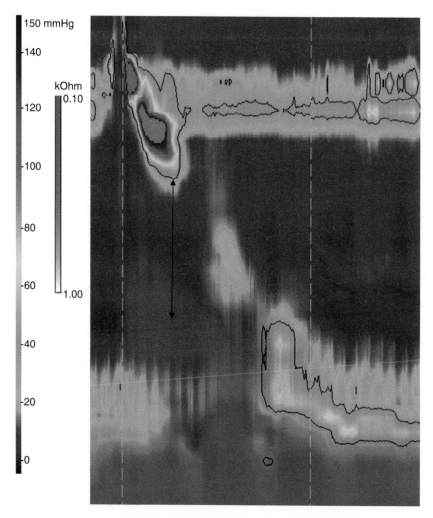

Figure 2.44 High-resolution esophageal manometry with impedance: Fragmented peristalsis. The UES opens normally with the onset of wet swallow, and the striated esophageal contraction is normal. There is a 9-cm break in the 20 mm Hg isobaric contour (*arrow*), consistent with a large break (>5 cm). The contraction vigor (DCI) is 458 mmHg.sec.cm. According to the Chicago Classification V3.0, the criteria for fragmented peristalsis (minor disorder of peristalsis) require that 50% or more of wet swallows have large breaks with normal DCI (450–8000 mmHg.sec.cm). Owing to the fragmented peristalsis, there is a "bolus escape" in the mid esophagus, consistent with incomplete bolus clearance

and proximal esophagus remains the primary tool in making the diagnosis, but as high-resolution esophageal manometry allows the continuous assessment of swallowing from hypopharynx to the proximal stomach, the HRM evaluation provides certain clues that may point to neuromuscular disorders in the striated esophagus and hypopharynx, such as cricopharyngeal bar and/or Zenker's diverticulum.

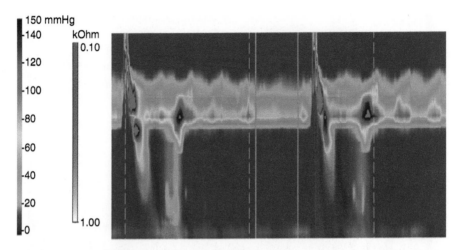

Figure 2.45 High-resolution esophageal manometry with impedance in a patient with oropharyngeal dysphagia. This zoomed-in view focuses on the upper part of the esophagus, where pooling of salt water is seen in the epiglottic valleculae. This impedance finding could explain the patient's recurrent cough and throat clearing, with an increased risk of aspiration and pneumonia. Patients with oropharyngeal dysphagia require further workup, including a videofluoroscopic swallowing study and an assessment by a speech language pathologist using specialized tests, including a volume viscous swallowing test, cough test, and 3-ounce water swallow test. Neurologic conditions such as stroke or Parkinson's disease could manifest with this type of presentation

On esophageal fluoroscopy, a cricopharyngeal bar is seen as a posterior indentation of the cricopharyngeal muscle on the cervical esophagus. In studies with both videofluoroscopy and esophageal manometry, a cricopharyngeal bar is not associated with impaired UES relaxation, but rather is characterized by decreased cricopharyngeal muscle compliance; the cricopharyngeus muscle does not distend normally during swallowing. The HRM often shows an elevated intrabolus pressure above the UES (Fig. 2.46), which may be a compensatory mechanism in response to flow across the UES.

Zenker's diverticulum is a pseudodiverticulum (mucosal pouch) seen as a herniation through an area of weakness in a region known as Killian's triangle. This area is formed by the cricopharyngeus muscle and the inferior pharyngeal constrictor muscle. A Zenker's diverticulum results from increased hypopharyngeal pressure due to stiffening of the cricopharyngeus muscle or age-related decreased elasticity of the tissue. The diverticulum can coexist with a cricopharyngeal bar. Dynamic esophageal fluoroscopy or an esophagogram remains the gold standard for diagnosis. Endoscopy has a limited role in identifying Zenker's diverticulum, as the opening may not be readily seen. Currently, there is no manometric reference to reliably identify a Zenker's diverticulum on HRM. Normal relaxation but incomplete opening of cricopharyngeus muscle may be seen; this high intrabolus pressure may result in a pulsion diverticulum. Sometimes a "double contour" can

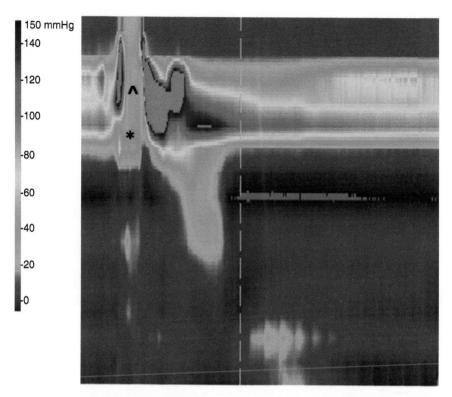

Figure 2.46 High-resolution esophageal manometry of cricopharyngeal bar (CPB). In this zoomed-in view of the upper part of the esophagus, the UES does not fully relax (*asterisk*) with the onset of the wet swallow, and its pressure does not equal the proximal esophageal pressure, because of a cricopharyngeal bar (CPB), a prominence of the cricopharyngeal muscle. There is an increase in intrabolus pressure (*arrowhead*) proximal to the CPB, due to increased resistance to normal bolus flow. The patient may have oropharyngeal dysphagia. A barium esophagogram, which has a higher sensitivity to detect CPB, should be considered to correlate with the manometric findings

be seen at the UES pressure zone (Fig. 2.47). Impedance may show bolus retention just proximal to the UES. In patients with esophageal diverticula (e.g. Zenker's, epiphrenic, Killian-Jamieson or traction diverticulum), extra caution should be used during catheter insertion, as the tip of the catheter can be caught inside the diverticulum, and further advancement could cause perforation. Resistance in advancement of the catheter after it traverses the UES may be felt, with intensive nausea and heaving.

The bottom line is that esophageal manometry generally does not change the management of patients with oropharyngeal dysphagia. It can provide a quantitative evaluation of UES pressures and pharyngeal and striated esophagus contractions implicated in some neuromuscular disorders, and the role of high-resolution esophageal manometry is evolving in the ENT world.

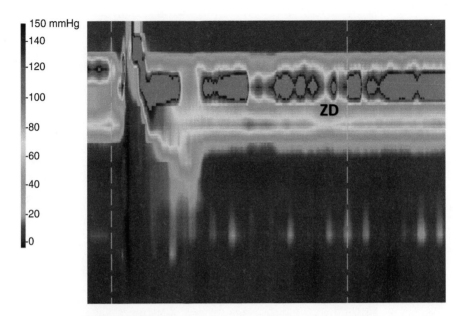

Figure 2.47 High-resolution esophageal manometry of Zenker's diverticulum (ZD). A ZD is a pseudodiverticulum due to a herniation through the Killian triangle, with the inferior pharyngeal constrictor bordering it superiorly and the cricopharyngeus muscle (CP) located inferiorly. The herniation is due to an increase in hypopharynx pressure secondary to CP stiffness or fibrosis, a hypertensive UES, or discoordination between the UES and the hypopharynx. It may coexist with a cricopharyngeal bar. Normally, the UES shows a single high-pressure band at rest, but this plot (which is zoomed in on the upper part of the esophagus) shows two areas of high pressure—a "double contour." The lower-pressure zone, shown in green between the two higher-pressure zones, corresponds to the diverticulum cavity. Given the 1-cm gap between the pressure sensors of the manometry catheter, esophageal HRM is less sensitive than a barium study in evaluating ZD

Hiatal Hernia

The phrenoesophageal ligaments anchor the diaphragm to the distal esophagus. The insertion point is approximately at the level of the squamocolumnar junction of the esophagus. During swallowing, the configuration of the whole apparatus changes, as the esophagus is shortened with longitudinal muscle contractions; in turn, the phrenoesophageal ligaments are stretched. This change is referred to as "physiologic hernia," as the gastric cardia is pulled caudally through the diaphragmatic hiatus with each swallow.

With the repetitive stress of swallowing over time, as well as other stressors such as increasing intra-abdominal pressure with recurrent vomiting, increased abdominal girth (i.e., obesity), pregnancy, etc., the phrenoesophageal membrane is subjected to substantial wear and tear. In addition, tonic esophageal longitudinal muscle contractions due to GERD and mucosal acidification may further disrupt this membrane, so that it may no longer be strong enough to maintain the distal esophagus in its normal anatomical position within the diaphragmatic hiatus. The result is herniation of the content of the abdominal cavity.

The gastroesophageal junction is a complex system, with a valvular mechanism partly attributable to the distal esophagus and proximal stomach, and partly to the crural diaphragmatic contractions. The compromised mechanisms in a hiatal hernia make those affected prone to developing pathological gastroesophageal reflux.

Hiatal hernias are broadly categorized into two classes—sliding hernias and paraesophageal hernias—but comprehensively, there are four types of hiatal hernias: Type I or sliding hiatal hernia is recognized by the displacement of gastroesophageal (GE) junction above the diaphragm, while the stomach remains in its normal anatomical position with the fundus below the GE junction. Types II to IV, which are subtypes of paraesophageal hernias, are true hernias with a hernia sac. A type II paraesophageal hernia is characterized by upward movement of the gastric fundus through the diaphragmatic hiatus, while the GE junction remains fixed to the arcuate ligament and preaortic fascia. A type III paraesophageal hernia is the combination of types I and II, in which both the GE junction and gastric fundus herniate caudally through the diaphragmatic hiatus, and the gastric fundus is above the GE junction. The type IV paraesophageal hernia occurs when the gastric fundus and another intra-abdominal organ (e.g., colon, small intestine, spleen, pancreas) herniate through a large defect in the phrenoesophageal membrane.

To measure a sliding hiatal hernia manometrically, the location of the LES and the diaphragmatic crural pinch are identified. The crural diaphragm is more easily identified when the patient is asked to take a deep breath, leading to crural contraction and a drop in the intra-esophageal pressure. The gap between the LES and the crural diaphragm allows the interpreter to estimate the size of the sliding hiatal hernia (Fig. 2.48).

The paraesophageal hernias are less often seen on HRM. Bolus accumulation in the paraesophageal hernia sac may be seen on esophageal impedance. If the paraesophageal hernia is large, it could cause manometric findings similar to that of EGJOO, as the hernia sac compresses the distal esophagus externally. Therefore, it is important to obtain a barium esophagogram to better delineate the anatomy of the esophagogastric junction, especially to confirm paraesophageal hernias.

Gastroesophageal Reflux Disease and Lower Esophageal Sphincter

According to the Montreal definition [7], GERD is present when there are bothersome symptoms and/or complications with the reflux of gastric content into the esophagus. Many factors contribute to the pathophysiology of GERD. As outlined earlier, the high-pressure zone in the distal esophagus is a complex entity, composed of the true LES and the crural diaphragm. Both these structures contribute to the integrity of the gastroesophageal sphincter. Therefore, in the setting of a hiatal hernia, where the optimal function of this complex zone is compromised, patients are more prone to developing GERD.

The LES is a segment of the tonically contracted smooth muscle in the GE junction. In a minority of patients with GERD, the LES resting pressure is diminished to less than 5 mm Hg. This in turn compromises the reflux barrier and makes it easy for the gastric pressure to overcome the LES pressure, leading to a retrograde reflux of gastric contents into the esophagus. Exogenous factors that may reduce the LES

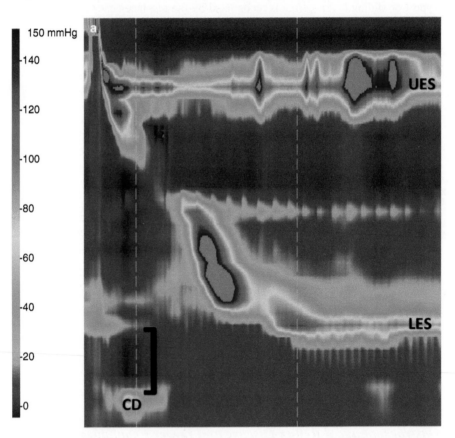

Figure 2.48 High-resolution esophageal manometry with impedance: Epiphrenic diverticulum and a large sliding hiatal hernia. A, The wet swallow results in normal esophageal primary peristalsis, and the LES relaxes normally with the onset of the swallow. The *bracket* marks a large hiatal hernia with diaphragmatic contraction seen 6 cm distal to the LES. **B,** The epiphrenic diverticulum is appreciated on impedance, as the fluid continuously pools in the diverticulum (*asterisk*). The diverticulum prevents the bolus from clearing the esophagus. The manometric finding should be correlated with an esophageal barium study and endoscopic evaluation. **C,** Barium esophagogram of the epiphrenic diverticulum (*asterisk*) and large sliding hiatal hernia (*double asterisks*). The *orange line* shows the diaphragmatic pinch distal to the hiatal hernia sac. Epiphrenic diverticula may be seen in patients with esophageal dysmotility

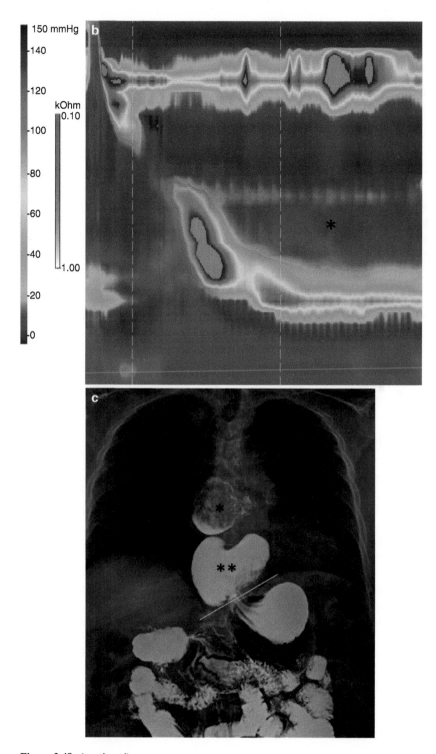

Figure 2.48 (continued)

resting pressure include high-fat meals, certain medications (e.g., calcium channel blockers, beta agonists, anticholinergics, nitrates), and habits such as smoking. Endogenous hormones such as nitric oxide, progesterone, and cholecystokinin also have a similar effect. In addition, the esophageal dysmotility associated with connective tissue disorders such as scleroderma can diminish the LES resting pressure and increase the risk of severe GERD and reflux esophagitis.

Transient LES Relaxation (TLESR)

Many GERD patients in fact have a normal LES resting pressure. The LES normally relaxes transiently in response to swallowing and proximal gastric distension; this is a vagally mediated reflex. When the number of occurrences of transient LES relaxation (TLESR) increases inappropriately, the individual can develop GERD (Fig. 2.49). The increased frequency of TLESRs is in fact the most common mechanism in the pathophysiology of GERD.

Finally, there are several barrier mechanisms that assist in esophageal clearance and "housekeeping" to rid the esophagus of any residual food bolus, as the severity of reflux damage is proportional to the acid exposure time. Impaired saliva production, diminished esophageal mucosal resistance, underlying esophageal dysmotility with impaired primary and secondary peristalsis, and gastroparesis may all contribute to worsening GERD.

Esophageal Dysmotility in Connective Tissue Disorders

Many connective tissue disorders have GI manifestations. In fact, the esophagus is one of the most commonly involved organs. For example, patients with systemic sclerosis, a multisystem autoimmune condition, are known to have skin involvement and various GI symptoms. Patients often complain of GERD, regurgitation, dysphagia, abdominal pain, nausea, vomiting, early satiety, diarrhea, or constipation. On the esophageal HRM, patients have a hypotensive LES, ineffective esophageal motility, absent peristalsis in the smooth muscle esophagus with intact striated esophageal contractions, and failed provocative tests (such as multiple rapid swallows), although some patients may have normal HRM. Rarely, other conditions such as achalasia can also be seen, but it is not specific to any connective tissue disorder [8].

Other connective tissue disorders, such as Sjögren's syndrome, CREST, overlap syndrome, polymyositis, dermatomyositis, and systemic lupus erythematosus may also have similar esophageal dysmotility. Figures 2.50 and 2.51 show examples.

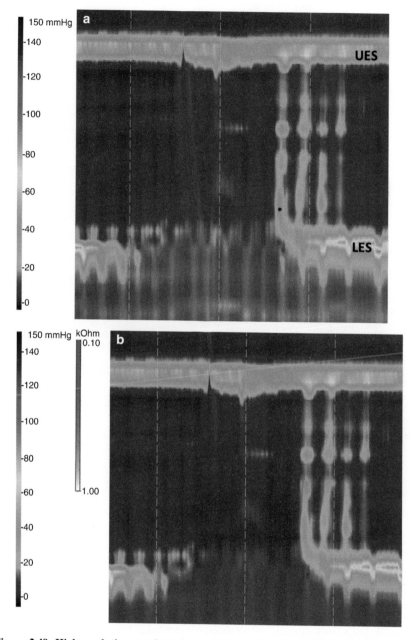

Figure 2.49 High-resolution esophageal manometry of transient LES relaxation. A, This study shows an 18-second interval of LES relaxation, demonstrated by the absence of LES resting pressure. The return of the LES resting pressure to baseline is followed by secondary contractions (*asterisk*), an appropriate response to TLESR. See also a very brief disruption in the UES resting pressure, as the subject takes a small dry swallow with no subsequent primary peristalsis. **B,** The same HRM with impedance makes it easy to appreciate the reflux of gastric content during the TLESR. The secondary contractions ensue to clear the esophagus of any refluxate

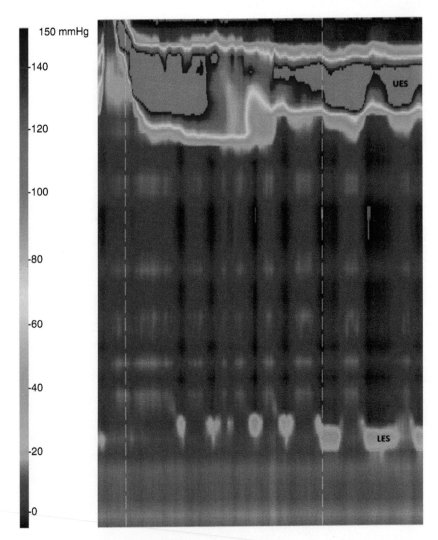

Figure 2.50 High-resolution esophageal manometry: Effects of a connective tissue disorder.
Aperistalsis in the mid and distal esophagus and significantly low LES resting pressure are findings
classically seen in patients with scleroderma or other connective tissue disorders. Absent contractility based on the Chicago Classification V3.0 requires 100% failed peristalsis, as seen in this
study, with normal integrated resting pressure in LES (i.e., IRP ≤15 mm Hg). In fact, the LES
resting pressure is almost completely due to diaphragmatic contraction, as seen with the crural
diaphragmatic contraction, which coincides with the inspiratory phase. Note that the proximal striated esophagus is intact. The UES resting pressure is elevated at 155 mm Hg, but the UES relaxation pressure is normal. The rise in UES resting pressure may be due to the catheter irritation or
the patient's anxiety or gagging during the esophageal manometry. Other differentials include
cervical osteophytes, thyromegaly, or (rarely) tumors of the head and neck

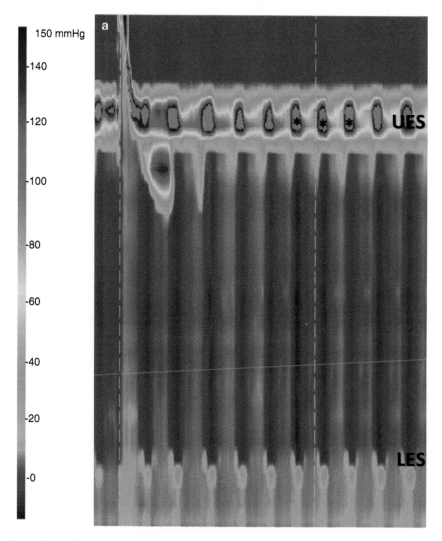

Figure 2.51 High-resolution esophageal manometry of scleroderma. A, A normal peristaltic contraction in the proximal striated esophagus follows wet swallows by this patient with scleroderma, but there is no esophageal peristalsis in the mid or distal esophagus. The LES resting pressure is negligible. These manometric findings increase GERD in scleroderma and can manifest as sore throat, voice hoarseness, heartburn, regurgitation, dysphagia, and increased risk of aspiration. This patient also has severe restrictive lung disease, manifested as tachypnea, "respiratory tugs" (*asterisks*) due to use of accessory muscles for breathing, and accentuated intrathoracic pressure variation between inspiration and expiration. **B,** Impedance highlights the lack of clearance of saline due to aperistaltic esophagus

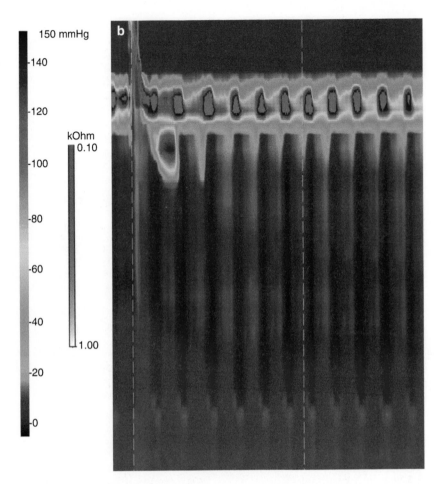

Figure 2.51   (continued)

Proximal Esophageal Dysmotility

The differential diagnoses for oropharyngeal or transfer dysphagia is quite broad: neurologic disorders, including stroke; neurodegenerative diseases, such as Parkinson's disease, progressive supranuclear palsy, multiple sclerosis, amyotrophic lateral sclerosis, Wilson's disease, and autonomic neuropathy (including Guillain-Barre syndrome); or neuromuscular junction disorders such as myasthenia gravis. In addition, myopathic disorders (such as hereditary myotonic dystrophy) or acquired myopathies such as polymyositis or dermatomyositis could present with similar symptoms, and patients with head and neck surgery who undergo radiation may have esophageal muscle weakness that is noticeable in hypopharyngeal, UES, and striated esophageal muscles (Fig. 2.52). Therefore, it is pertinent to obtain a thorough history prior to performing additional investigations such as dynamic, video-assisted esophageal fluoroscopy and HRM.

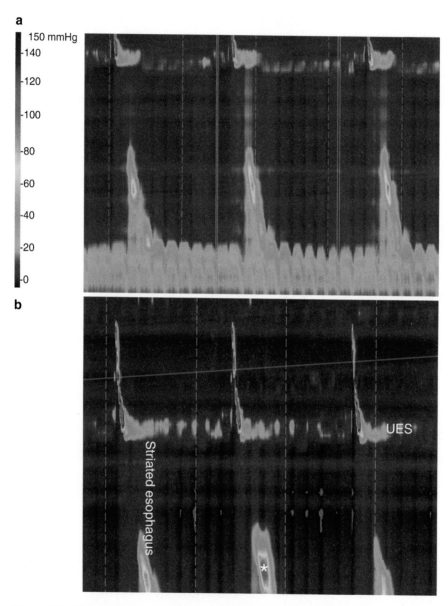

Figure 2.52 High-resolution esophageal manometry after head and neck radiation therapy.
A, The UES resting pressure is quite diminished, measuring 2.7 mm Hg; normal is 34–104 mm Hg.
In addition, the proximal striated esophagus does not contract with the onset of wet swallows. The
distal esophagus is not affected by head and neck radiation, so the peristaltic contraction is intact
and propagates normally. Given the low UES resting pressure and the absence of contraction in the
striated esophagus, these patients are at increased risk of aspiration. **B,** In this zoomed-in view of
the hypopharynx and proximal esophagus after radiation therapy, HRM shows that the hypopharynx (the base of the tongue and velopharynx) contracts normally, but the UES resting pressure is
significantly low. The UES relaxes normally; therefore, there is no significant fibrosis/stenosis that
could impair the UES relaxation. Finally, the proximal striated esophagus does not contract with
the wet swallows, due to the effect of the radiation therapy. The beginning of the normal smooth
muscle contraction of the mid esophagus is noted (*asterisk*)

Classically, disorders such as myasthenia gravis present with dysphagia and bulbar symptoms (for example, jaw muscle weakness, dysphagia, nasal regurgitation, dysphonia, dysarthria). On HRM, patients have a diminished UES resting pressure, and the proximal striated esophagus is predominantly affected. Striated muscle myopathies can rarely affect the smooth muscle esophagus as well, but more importantly, fatigability may become pronounced with sequential swallows or provocative testing. Therefore, a history of bulbar symptoms and fatigability, and an improvement of symptoms in response to anti-cholinesterase inhibitors may be quite valuable in the diagnosis of striated esophageal dysmotility on HRM.

Myotonic dystrophy (Figs. 2.53–2.55) is a heterogenous hereditary condition associated with skeletal muscle weakness, myotonic contractions, cardiac conduction abnormalities, cataract, and other abnormalities.

Esophageal Diverticula

By definition, a diverticulum is an abnormal pouch, which is usually believed to be due to abnormal pressure along the GI tract. In the esophagus, the Killian's triangle (as discussed earlier) is a weak pressure point in the hypopharynx. Posterior herniation of the mucosa in the Killian's triangle results in formation of a Zenker's

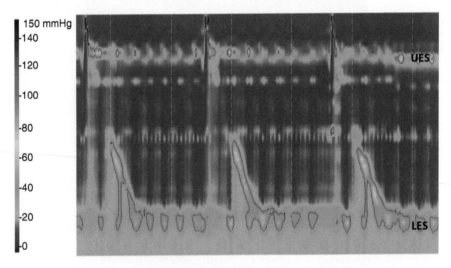

Figure 2.53 High-resolution esophageal manometry of myotonic dystrophy type I. Myotonic dystrophy is a clinically and genetically heterogeneous disorder with multisystem nature, causing skeletal muscle weakness, cataracts, cardiac conduction abnormalities, infertility, insulin resistance, and developmental delay. In this figure, the UES baseline pressure is low at 30 mm Hg. The proximal striated esophageal contractions are faintly present but are quite weak. There are large breaks, defined as a gap between the striated esophageal contraction and the onset of smooth muscle contraction, seen on the isobaric pressure contour of 20 mm Hg. The distal smooth muscle esophagus has peristaltic contractions, although with a weaker contraction vigor than normal (DCI, 300–400 mmHg.sec.cm), so the contractions are accounted as weak peristalsis rather than fragmented contraction, which requires minimum contraction vigor of 450 mmHg.sec.cm. The IRP is normal

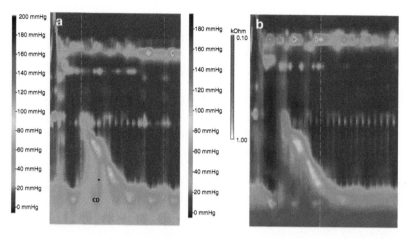

Figure 2.54 High-resolution esophageal manometry of an isolated wet swallow of myotonic dystrophy type I. A, The UES pressure is noticeably low, and the proximal striated esophageal contraction is quite weak. The distal esophagus produces a peristaltic contraction with near-normal contraction vigor. The LES resting pressure and its relaxation pressure are normal, and there are CD contractions with inspiration. Note the transient rise in the intrabolus pressure coinciding with the CD contractions (*asterisk*). **B,** High-resolution esophageal manometry with impedance shows "bolus escape" in the proximal esophagus, which is due to the lack of striated esophageal contraction. The impedance does not fully return to baseline, suggestive of incomplete bolus clearance

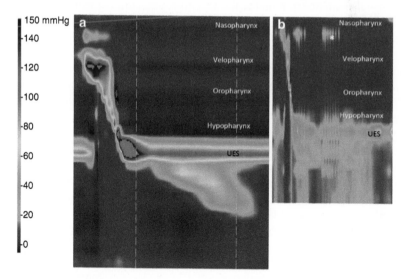

Figure 2.55 High-resolution manometry of the hypopharynx and the upper esophagus of patients with normal HRM (A) and myotonic dystrophy (B). The velopharynx is a muscular valve consisting of the lateral and posterior pharyngeal walls and the soft palate, essential in speech. With the onset of a swallow, the normal HRM shows a slight cephalic movement of the soft palate, followed by a diagonal propagation of contraction. The UES opens with the onset of wet swallows, and it returns to its baseline pressure after the bolus passes through. In contrast, when the patient with myotonic dystrophy is asked to say "KaKaKa" (*asterisk*), contractions are seen and reflected along the UES, but they are relatively weak. The UES relaxes normally in response to a wet swallow. The proximal striated esophageal contraction is also noted to be weak

diverticulum. Unlike Zenker's, which is a posterior and inferior herniation through the Killian's triangle, the less common Killian's diverticulum is an anterolateral herniation at the level of C5–C6 vertebrae; it is due to a congenital weakness of the cervical esophagus below the level of the cricopharyngeus muscle. Killian's diverticulum is often asymptomatic.

Thoracic esophageal diverticula are relatively uncommon. Patients may be asymptomatic or present with chest pain, food regurgitation, GERD, dysphagia, or weight loss. Most patients with this condition have esophageal motility disorders such as achalasia. These diverticula are not as easily appreciated on esophageal manometry and may require ancillary tests such as barium esophagogram, upper endoscopy, or chest CT scans to delineate the anatomy, as seen in Figure 2.48. On HRM with impedance, the diverticulum pouch may be appreciated from the fluid accumulation in the sac. The HRM is important in diagnosing the underlying esophageal dysmotility leading to the diverticula formation in the first place.

Evaluation Before or after Peroral Endoscopic Myotomy (POEM) for Disorders of EGJ Outflow Obstruction

Esophageal manometry remains the essential preoperative evaluation for subjects undergoing endoscopic or surgical intervention for the major motility disorders, such as achalasia. Traditionally, pneumatic dilation or Heller myotomy were the treatment options for patients with achalasia, but in 2010, peroral endoscopic myotomy (POEM) was introduced as an alternative to conventional Heller myotomy for the management of achalasia, with purportedly less morbidity and faster recovery time. However, the debate about superiority is still ongoing.

During POEM, a mucosal incision is made, followed by a submucosal tunnel traversing the EGJ, with subsequent myotomy. The mucosal incision is then closed with an endoscopic clip or suture. This technique is more widely used for achalasia, but it has also been reported in EGJ outflow obstruction and DES. Esophageal HRM provides valuable details for POEM planning, as the exact muscular segment involved in achalasia can be targeted with a more precise length of required myotomy, individualizing this endoscopic approach to each achalasia subject.

Figure 2.56 shows an HRM of a patient with dysphagia who was found to have achalasia type II. The patient underwent POEM, but she developed recurrent symptoms after POEM (Fig. 2.57). Therefore, the esophageal manometry was repeated. The repeat study showed persistent segment of spastic contraction (Fig. 2.58), which was likely unmasked with the post-POEM improvement in the panesophageal pressurization pattern in achalasia II. She was referred for redo POEM, with targeted myotomy of the involved spastic segment, and subsequently reported improvement of her symptoms.

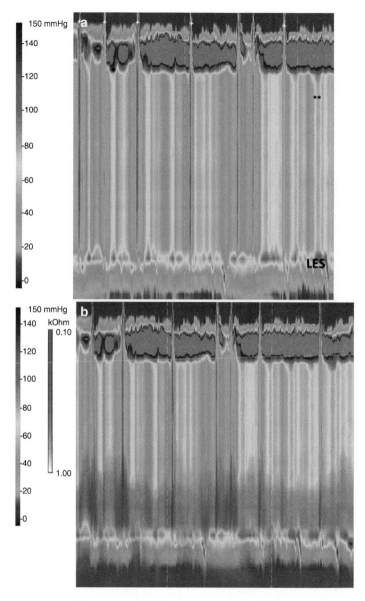

Figure 2.56 High-resolution esophageal manometry of achalasia type II with panesophageal pressurization. **A,** The striated proximal esophagus generates peristaltic contraction (*asterisk*) with the onset of wet swallows, but there is no peristaltic contraction along the rest of the esophagus, demonstrated by the absence of diagonal bands of pressure. Multiple wet swallows (*plus signs*) led to simultaneous, repetitive panesophageal pressurization, as demonstrated by vertical columns of high pressure along the entire length of the esophagus. Note also the secondary panesophageal pressurization (*double asterisks*). Generally, the contraction vigor of panesophageal pressurizations varies from one swallow to another during a study, but given the panesophageal pressurization, the DCI is not calculated. The LES does not relax in response to wet swallows, as demonstrated by increased IRP of 60 mm Hg (normal IRP is <15 mm Hg). These criteria indicate a diagnosis of achalasia type II. **B,** Because of the absence of normal LES relaxation, impedance shows that the bolus does not clear the esophagus. The accumulation of normal saline with its electrolytes conducts electrical current between the impedance sensors and decreases impedance, as demonstrated by the purple hue

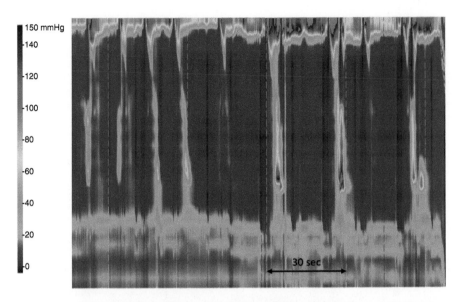

Figure 2.57 High-resolution esophageal manometry of the patient in Figure 2.56 after per-oral endoscopic myotomy (POEM). The patient underwent POEM with the posterior entry approach. A mucosal tunnel was made at 27 cm from the incisors, and subsequently the gastro-scope was advanced into the tunnel, and a submucosal incision was made that allowed endoscopic circular myotomy from 32 cm all the way through the GE junction at 43 cm. Two months later, the patient developed recurrent dysphagia, although milder than the initial presentation. This repeat HRM was obtained, showing an improvement in the LES resting pressure, which decreased from 71 mm Hg to 18 mm Hg (*not shown*). Mean IRP decreased from 60 mm Hg to 12 mm Hg. The first four swallows show premature contractions, (DL: 3.2 sec), with a high-pressure zone from 28 cm to 38 cm, which may be due to post-POEM granulation tissue or an inadequate cir-cular myotomy during POEM. Upper endoscopy ruled out granulation tissue, so the high-pres-sure zone in the mid esophagus is most likely due to an inadequate circular myotomy. This manifestation is further pronounced with the provocative testing, which in this case was with salt cracker (final 3 swallows). This manometric study curiously suggests that achalasia type II has regressed to type III post-POEM

Evaluation Before or after Nissen Fundoplication

The Nissen fundoplication is one of the surgical treatments for GERD, used if medi-cal therapy fails or causes adverse effects, or if the patient wishes to avoid long-term use of a PPI or H_2 receptor antagonist (H_2RA). In the Nissen fundoplication, which is usually performed laparoscopically, the gastric fundus is wrapped 360 degrees around the LES to strengthen the sphincter, prevent acid reflux, and allow repair of the sliding hiatal hernia. Other surgical approaches include a partial wrap such as a Toupet fundoplication (a 270-degree wrap on the posterior side) or a Dor fundopli-cation (180-degree wrap on the anterior side). Other technologies, such as a laparo-scopic magnetic barrier (LINX®, developed by Torax Medical Inc.) have been used in place of the Nissen fundoplication, promising less invasive surgery, faster recov-ery, and fewer side effects, including less "bloat-man syndrome," experienced by

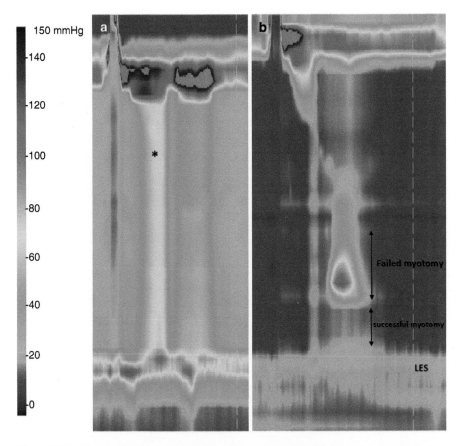

Figure 2.58 High-resolution esophageal manometry of achalasia type II before and after POEM. A, Loss of inhibitory noncholinergic (nitric oxide–producing) neurons leads to aperistalsis and panesophageal pressurization (*asterisk*), as evident by a vertical column of high pressure, extending the entire length of the esophagus. Normally, the inhibitory neurons innervating the esophageal smooth muscles are first activated to relax the esophagus, in order to promote esophageal filling and bolus transit, facilitated by nitric oxide release. This is followed by the activation of cholinergic excitatory neurons, to promote peristalsis. Loss of the balance between inhibitory innervation and excitatory neurons in achalasia results in an inappropriate increase in the resting LES pressure and prevents the LES from relaxing normally with the onset of a wet swallow. **B,** After POEM, there is a regression of the achalasia type II to achalasia type III, as shown by a premature contraction in the distal esophagus (DL: 3.2 sec), which is due to a failed POEM with inadequate disruption of the circular muscle in the mid-esophagus. However, the IRP shows an improvement after the POEM procedure

those who are unable to belch post-Nissen. However, capsular adhesions around the LINX® device have been reported; these could encapsulate the vagus nerve and cause adverse events such as dysphagia, esophageal dysmotility, gastroparesis, and nausea.

Figure 2.59 shows some examples of manometric findings before and after Nissen fundoplication, illustrating potential postoperative complications.

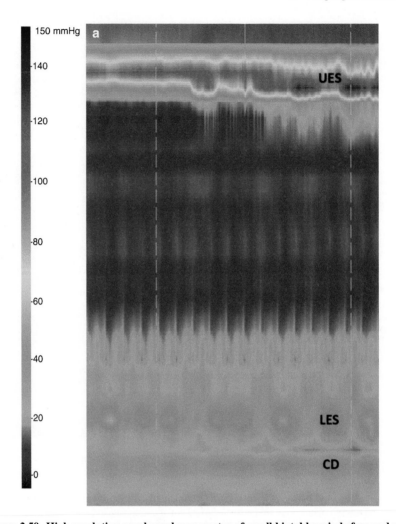

Figure 2.59 High-resolution esophageal manometry of small hiatal hernia before and after Nissen fundoplication. A, The UES appears as a band of high pressure proximally. At rest, the UES remains closed. The LES and the CD generate two areas of high-pressure zones distally. Normally, the LES and CD generate a single, juxtaposed area of high pressure in the distal esophagus in the region of the GE junction. In this HRM, however, these two bands are separated by 2.5 cm, implying that there is a 2.5-cm sliding hiatal hernia. The respiratory cycle variation above the CD shows a decrease in pressure on inspiration and an increase in pressure with expiration, a cycle opposite to what is seen below the CD, in the abdominal cavity. Therefore, the pressure inversion point (PIP) is along the CD. This confirms the presence of a 2.5-cm sliding hiatal hernia. **B,** HRM of the same patient after Nissen fundoplication. The previously seen 2.5-cm sliding hiatal hernia is seen again here, suggesting that the Nissen fundoplication is disrupted. **C,** In the same patient, HRM with impedance shows that the bolus clears the esophagus initially with the primary peristalsis, but because of the failed Nissen wrap, the patient has reflux, as seen by retrograde bolus movement from the stomach into the mid esophagus

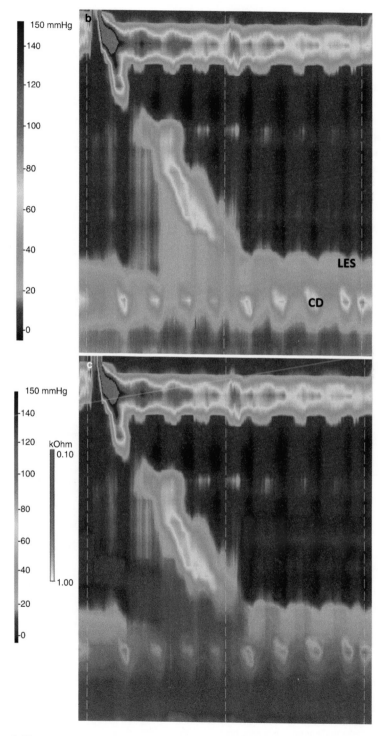

Figure 2.59 (continued)

Evaluation of Belching

The retrograde passage of esophageal or gastric gas out of the mouth is referred to as *belching* or *eructation*. According to the Rome IV criteria, belching disorder is divided into two sub-types, depending on the origin of the refluxate: *supragastric belch* is a habitual disorder with repetitive aerophagia and recurrent belching. The air enters the esophagus and often exits it shortly after, without entering the stomach (Fig. 2.60). On the other hand, *gastric belching* occurs when gastric air is eructated (Fig. 2.61). Esophageal venting, with LES and UES relaxation, can be a response to filling of the esophagus; examples of esophageal venting are seen throughout these chapters.

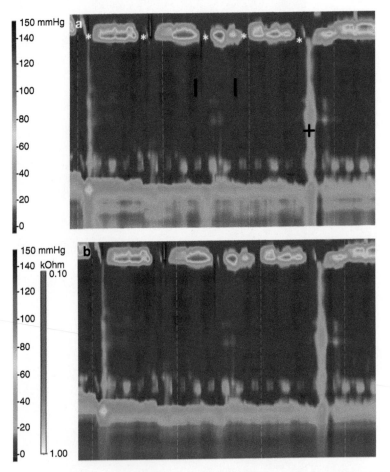

Figure 2.60 High-resolution esophageal manometry and impedance of aerophagia. A, Shown are repetitive relaxations of the UES (*asterisks*), which are preceded by deep inspiration (I). The deep inspiration makes intrathoracic pressure more negative, which creates a vacuum effect, leading to aboral air entry into the esophagus. This is a behavioral pattern seen in subjects with aerophagia and supragastric belch. After multiple episodes of aerophagia, the subject belches (*plus sign*), as evident by rise in the intragastric pressure to eject the swallowed air. As there is no LES relaxation, this is likely a supragastric belch. **B,** The HRM with impedance in the same subject shows no drop in the impedance with the episodes of aerophagia, suggesting that there is no associated reflux

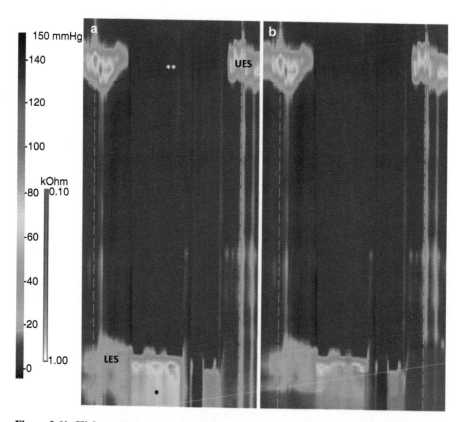

Figure 2.61 High-resolution esophageal manometry with impedance: A long, 8-second gastric belch. A, There is an increase in the intra-gastric pressure, which overcomes the LES pressure. There is no significant retrograde fluid regurgitation in the esophagus, but the belch could have led to retrograde movement of air, which may not generate high-pressure columns in the esophagus. The UES relaxes (*double asterisks*) to expel air, and then returns to baseline at the end of the belch. **B,** HRM with impedance of the same belch allows better evaluation of the belch content. The fluid regurgitation is associated with a drop in impedance; air has higher impedance. The impedance did not change from baseline, which suggests the belch was solely gas, rather than fluid

Belching can be seen on esophageal manometry as a non–swallow-related decrease in the UES resting pressure, which allows the esophagus to expel air. Differentiating between supragastric and gastric belching often requires pH-impedance. The approach to interpreting pH-impedance is further covered in Chapter 5.

Evaluation of Rumination Syndrome

Once thought to be a behavioral condition occurring in mentally challenged patients, it is now recognized that rumination syndrome can occur in otherwise healthy individuals [9]. It is characterized by spontaneous regurgitation of recently ingested food, which is due to an unintentional but voluntary intragastric pressure rise greater than 30 mm Hg, generated by contractions of the abdominal wall muscles. Once this pressure overcomes the LES pressure, the gastric content flows in the esophagus and then the mouth; then it is either spat out or remasticated. This diagnosis should be differentiated from GERD, especially in patients with "PPI-refractory GERD." The diagnosis of rumination syndrome should be considered when there is a reflux event extending to the proximal esophagus that is associated with an increase in abdominal pressure greater than 30 mm Hg shortly after or during the feeding phase.

Three distinct subtypes are recognized: *Primary rumination* occurs without any triggers (Fig. 2.62). *Secondary rumination* is similar to primary rumination but is preceded by an episode of reflux. Finally, *supragastric belching–associated rumination syndrome* starts with a decline in intrathoracic pressure (precipitated by transient diaphragmatic contraction) and aboral movement of air bolus in the esophagus due to the "vacuum effect" generated by a further drop in esophageal pressure during deep inspiration. The air is then forcefully expelled upward in the esophagus, owing to the rise in intragastric pressure; subsequent retrograde movement of gastric contents ensues (Fig. 2.63).

Rumination syndrome often requires prolonged HRM evaluation (30–90 minutes in duration) with a standardized test meal or the subject's choice of provoking meal. This condition is indistinguishable from reflux episodes if it is only evaluated based on pH-impedance; it could be falsely labeled as pathologic reflux. Knowledge of

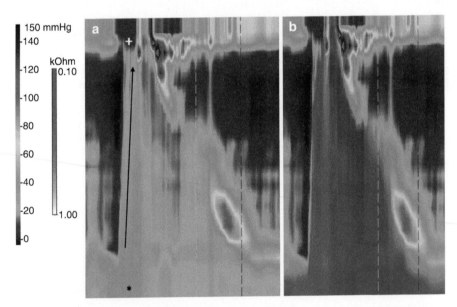

Figure 2.62 High-resolution esophageal manometry and impedance in a patient with primary rumination syndrome. A, Shortly after a provoking meal, the intragastric pressure rises to >30 mm Hg (*asterisk*). The pressure ultimately overcomes the LES resting pressure and causes the retrograde expulsion (*arrow*) of the gastric contents. This is followed by UES relaxation (*plus sign*) and subsequent swallowing of the regurgitant, which results in a normal primary peristaltic contraction. **B,** In the same patient, impedance makes it possible to differentiate between gas and liquid regurgitant. In this episode of rumination, liquid gastric content moves into the esophagus, but the primary peristalsis clears the esophagus of any residual bolus, and the impedance returns to baseline

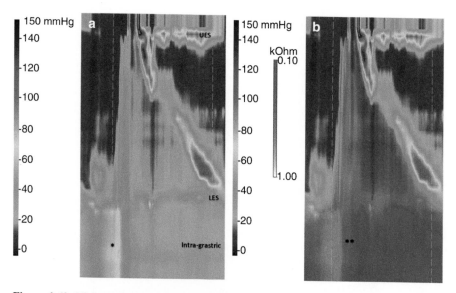

Figure 2.63 High-resolution esophageal manometry of supragastric belching–associated rumination syndrome. A, Rumination syndrome is a functional gastrointestinal disorder, characterized by effortless intra- or immediately post-prandial retrograde bolus movement. Manometrically, it is characterized by a transient increase in intragastric pressure (*asterisk*) greater than 30 mm Hg, which overcomes the LES resting pressure. The UES is initially closed, but it eventually opens, and the gastric content flows into the mouth. The intragastric pressure then returns to baseline. **B,** Impedance allows easier evaluation of bolus movement. With the increase in the gastric pressure, the gastric content is moved into the esophagus (*double asterisks*) and eventually into the hypopharynx. The patient can then spit out the gastric content or re-masticate and re-swallow it. In this case, the patient re-swallows the content and a primary peristalsis propagates along the entire length of the esophagus, clearing the bolus. Impedance returns to baseline at the end of the primary peristalsis

these behavioral disorders is the key to proceeding with appropriate tests, as patients with recurrent belching or rumination syndrome generally do not respond to PPI therapy. The mainstay of therapy is patient education, behavioral therapy with a speech language pathologist, diaphragmatic breathing, and stopping unnecessary PPIs.

High-Resolution Manometric Finding of Vomiting

Figure 2.64 shows HRM and impedance during an episode of vomiting.

Manometric Findings after Foregut Surgeries

HRM and impedance studies after foregut surgeries such as lap band or sleeve gastrectomy can reveal ongoing problems, and may provide guidance for further management plan (Figs. 2.65–2.68).

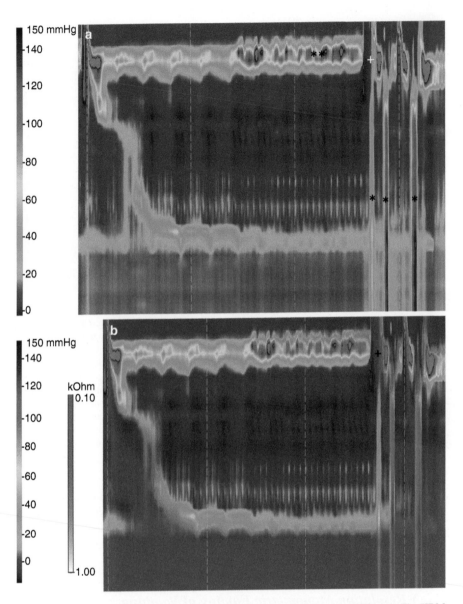

Figure 2.64 High-resolution esophageal manometry of an episode of vomiting. A, The HRM shows a wet swallow, resulting in a primary peristalsis. After 15 seconds, the UES pressure rises as patient becomes nauseated and anxious (*double asterisks*). Subsequently, after the second wet swallow (*plus sign*), three heaves/vomiting episodes occur, demonstrated by high-pressure columns (*asterisks*). The UES relaxes to expel the regurgitant. Note that vomiting is always followed by an immediate attempt to swallow, to minimize aspiration. **B,** The impedance allows better evaluation of the bolus movement. After the initial wet swallow, the bolus does completely clear the esophagus. With contraction of the abdominal muscles during heaving/vomiting, the bolus enters the esophagus and is partly expelled

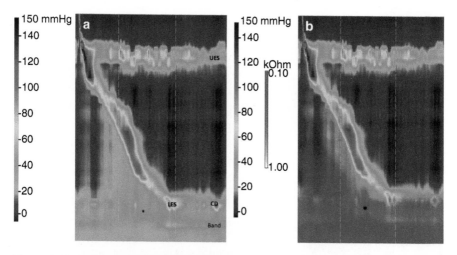

Figure 2.65 High-resolution esophageal manometry and impedance of normal gastric lap band. A, The UES relaxes normally in response to a wet swallow, and the wet swallow resulted in a normal peristaltic contraction. The LES relaxes with the onset of the wet swallow and it returns to the baseline pressure at the end of peristalsis. There is a second high-pressure band distal to the LES, consistent with the normal gastric lap band. The gap between the LES and gastric lap band corresponds to the small gastric pouch, which promotes early satiety in patients undergoing this bariatric surgery. **B,** The HRM with impedance does not show any obstruction to the bolus flow with the gastric lap band. There is mild pressurization in the gastric pouch during the wet swallow (*asterisk*), which is normal. The bolus clears the esophagus appropriately

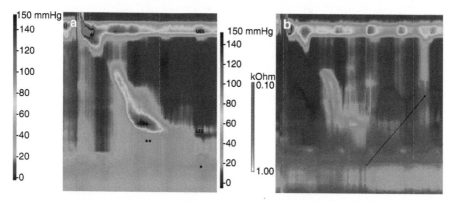

Figure 2.66 High-resolution esophageal manometry and impedance post–lap band: A large hiatal hernia. A, There is normal opening of the UES with the onset of swallow, followed by a normal primary esophageal peristalsis. The LES resting pressure is low. A horizontal band of high pressure represents a combination of the crural diaphragm and the lap band (*asterisk*). There is a large (6 cm) hiatal hernia, suggestive the lap band has slipped. There is pressurization in the hiatal sac (*double asterisks*), as the lap band generates a high-pressure zone that does not relax for the bolus to pass. **B,** The HRM with impedance shows lap band slip with a large hiatal hernia. The bolus transiently clears the esophagus into the intrathoracic gastric pouch/hiatal hernia, but at the end of the esophageal peristalsis, there is bolus accumulation in the hernia sac. Given the diminished resting LES pressure and presence of hernia, there is retrograde bolus movement into the mid esophagus (*arrow*)

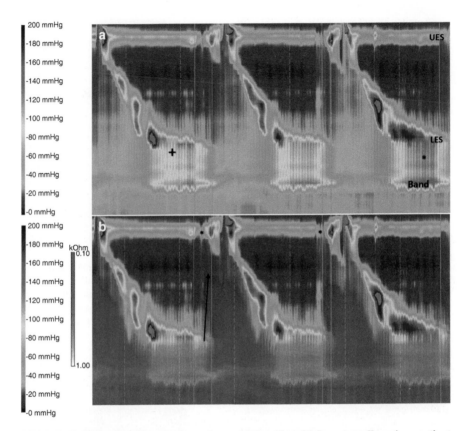

Figure 2.67 High-resolution esophageal manometry of multiple wet swallows in a patient with slipped gastric band. A, The wet swallows yielded three peristaltic contractions. The LES is in the thoracic cavity. A large hiatal hernia (*plus sign*) is seen. Because the band does not physiologically relax after onset of the swallow, it appears as a band of persistent pressure. With the onset of the swallow, the body of the esophagus is propagating the peristaltic contraction, which results in pressurization within the hiatal sac (*asterisk*), shown as columns of higher pressure. This pattern repeats itself on repetitive swallows, with increasing pressure in the hiatal sac, due to bolus accumulation above the slipped gastric band. **B,** HRM with impedance in the same patient shows that the bolus is retained in the hiatal sac, proximal to the band, owing to its persistently higher pressure. The subject belches (*asterisk*) to relieve the pressure in the esophagus, which results in the retrograde movement of the bolus (*arrow*), easily appreciated from the impedance. The incomplete clearance of the bolus after the second and third wet swallows is demonstrated by the persistent purple hue at the end of the peristaltic contractions

Troubleshooting

Table 2.1 lists a variety of technical problems that can arise during high-resolution manometry.

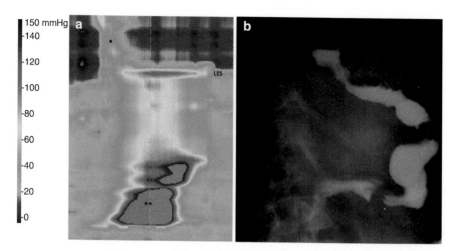

Figure 2.68 High-resolution esophageal manometry after sleeve gastrectomy. A, This image does not show the entire esophageal peristalsis, as the catheter was advanced 20 cm caudally into the remnant stomach. The *asterisk* shows the end of the primary esophageal peristalsis. There is pressurization in the proximal remnant stomach after entry of the bolus, owing to the stapled line of the sleeve gastrectomy. This is followed by a segment with higher pressure (*double asterisks*), a finding that corresponds to an angulation along the sleeve gastrectomy staple line, which was further verified on the barium study. **B,** The barium swallow in the same patient shows the sharp angulation along the distal sleeve gastrectomy staple line. The patient may present with regurgitation, nausea, vomiting, and associated weight loss. Endoluminal stenting could be considered to temporize symptoms, with more definitive surgical management to follow, such as Roux-en-Y

Inability to Intubate

At times, the catheter may encounter resistance as it is advanced through the nasal passages. This may be due to nasopharyngeal deformities such as deviated septum. It is important to advance the catheter slowly and try to negotiate it through curvatures of the nasal passage, but this may be quite challenging if deformities are severe. Both nares should be attempted for the catheter insertion. Applying adequate lubricant and topical anesthetics will generally ease the catheter insertion. The catheter should not be forced if there is significant resistance. If the insertion of the catheter is not technically feasible, then the catheter may be placed endoscopically or under fluoroscopic guidance, although this is more labor-intensive and requires post-procedural coordination to ensure that the sedation adequately wears off and it will not impact the result of the esophageal manometry. In addition, the placement of the catheter into the esophagus under endoscopy must be carried out carefully to avoid damaging the sensors.

Table 2.1 Troubleshooting of Technical Challenges in High-Resolution Manometry

Technical Challenge	Troubleshooting Methods
Allergy to lidocaine or history of methemoglobinemia	Use water-based lubricants instead of lidocaine
Difficulty with catheter insertion through nasal passage	Adequate catheter lubrication Assess anatomical malformation, such as deviated septum Trial of both nostrils Maintain the head in a neutral position to start Vertical insertion of the catheter to prevent catheter from being trapped between inferior and middle turbinates
Encountering resistance at UES	Chin tuck, head tilt down Sips of water to facilitate catheter passage through the UES Breathing through the nose to suppress the gagging sensation
Severe ear pain during insertion	Due to irritation of Eustachian tube by the catheter; withdraw the catheter and use the other nostril for reinsertion
Catheter enters oral cavity	Withdraw the catheter into the nasal passage Reinsert with chin tuck and head tilt down
Severe cough and/or inability to breathe	Withdraw the catheter to ensure it is not in the trachea May also occur due to laryngospasm: Withdraw the catheter, have the patient breathe slowly, and wait for a few minutes before reinsertion, if stable
Encountering resistance below UES	Confirm patient does not have esophageal diverticulum
Difficulty traversing the LES (e.g., achalasia)	Maintain an upright body posture Pull the catheter back to ensure it is straight Cautiously give small sips of water, while evaluating impedance for bolus clearance Advance the catheter when patient takes a deep inspiration and holds it Use carbonated drinks to induce esophageal vents, which relax the LES
Large hiatal hernia	Ensure catheter is straight Look for "butterfly-pattern" suggestive of folded catheter in hiatal hernia
Paraesophageal hernia	Prior knowledge of esophageal anatomy is helpful Keep catheter straight Ask patient to inspire deeply to assess catheter passage through the LES
Patient heaves and vomits	Use relaxation and reassurance techniques
Patient cannot stop swallowing	Instruct patient to keep mouth slightly open and breath through the mouth Use relaxation techniques Consider performing wet swallows first and then measure the baseline pressures
Epistaxis	Most often self-limited, easily controlled by applying pressure on the nose
Sore throat after the procedure	Self-limiting, lasts only a few hours Consume warm beverages
Patient on home oxygen	Provide oxygen via nasal cannulas during manometry Consider active pulse oximetry during the procedure

LES—lower esophageal sphincter; UES—upper esophageal sphincter.

Once the catheter passes the nasopharynx and reaches the hypopharynx, the patient may experience a gagging sensation. The patient is then asked to tilt his or her head down and take small sips of water to facilitate catheter passage through the UES. In the presence of a cricopharyngeal bar, Zenker's diverticulum, severe cervical kyphosis with osteophytes, or cervical orthopedic plates, further resistance may be encountered in traversing the UES. Generally, taking small sips of water promotes UES relaxation and facilitates the catheter passage. Caution should be practiced in elderly patients with known cricopharyngeal bar, Zenker's diverticulum, or neurodegenerative diseases with oropharyngeal dysphagia, because of a high risk of aspiration. Pulling back the catheter, straightening it, and reinserting it in a "chin-tucked" position may be successful.

The third resistance point may be at the level of the LES, especially in patients with major motility disorders such as achalasia and EGJ outflow obstruction, in whom the LES does not relax with wet swallows. The catheter should be straightened, and the patient can take small sips of water to facilitate the catheter advancement. The catheter needs to traverse the LES and enters the stomach to accurately estimate the LES resting pressure. Raising the head of the bed or asking the patient to sit up may allow gravity to pull the catheter into the stomach. As the LES does not relax in achalasia, the impedance should be followed during the catheter insertion, to ensure the column of fluid is not extending into the proximal esophagus, which could increase the risk of aspiration. Asking the patient to continue with dry swallowing should help with catheter insertion.

Finally, in patients with a large hiatal hernia, the catheter may not enter into the stomach, as it tends to curl in the large hiatal sac (Fig. 2.69). A "butterfly pattern" may be seen if the catheter is folded on itself. The catheter should be pulled back and straightened for reinsertion. If the catheter could not traverse the GE junction in the stomach, then it should be noted that the LES resting pressure may not be accurately measured manometrically, as the LES resting pressure is calculated relative to the gastric pressure. The same difficulty may be encountered in patients who have a large paraesophageal hernia, as the hernia sac causes extrinsic pressure in the distal esophagus, which makes catheter insertion challenging. Therefore, knowing the anatomy of the esophagus prior to manometry is quite helpful.

Folded Catheter

In some patients, such as those with a large hiatal hernia or achalasia, the catheter may fold back upon itself before entering the stomach, while a "butterfly pattern" may be seen manometrically (Fig. 2.70). Reinsertion should be attempted.

Broken Catheter Sleeve

Malfunctioning sensors may indicate that the catheter needs repair or replacement (Fig. 2.71).

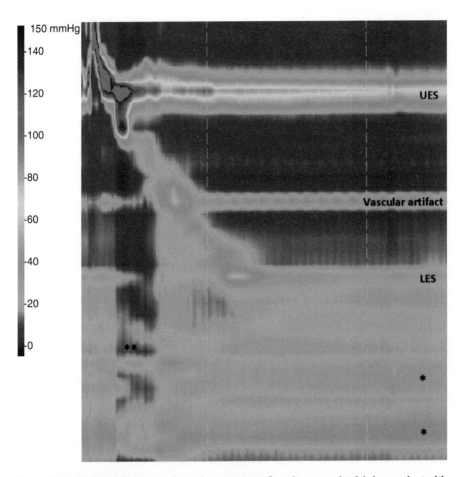

Figure 2.69   High-resolution esophageal manometry of a primary peristalsis in a patient with a massive sliding hiatal hernia. The LES is easily recognized after primary peristalsis. It is generally within 3 cm of the contraction deceleration point, where the slope of the primary peristalsis decreases in angulation, as the bolus enters the phrenic ampulla into the distal esophagus. The high-pressure band in mid esophagus appears to be pulsatile in nature. The catheter has not traversed the diaphragm, as the respiratory variations follow the same pattern along the catheter length below the LES as above the LES. There are two high-pressure bands (*asterisks*) distal to the LES, which represent the catheter curling in the large hiatal hernia sac, given the "butterfly/mirror-image pattern of both asterisks". As the catheter has not traversed into the stomach and is not straight, the accurate size of the hiatal hernia cannot be assessed manometrically. In addition, the LES resting pressure cannot be measured accurately, because it is measured relative to the gastric pressure, so the catheter must reach the intragastric lumen. If a patient is known to have a large hiatal hernia, it is often helpful to ask him or her to take a deep breath to appreciate the respiratory cycle variations above and below the diaphragm, to ensure that the catheter has crossed the PIP. In this study, the *double asterisks* show a deep inspiration, and the pressure pattern shows that the catheter remains in the intrathoracic cavity and has not crossed the diaphragm into the abdominal cavity

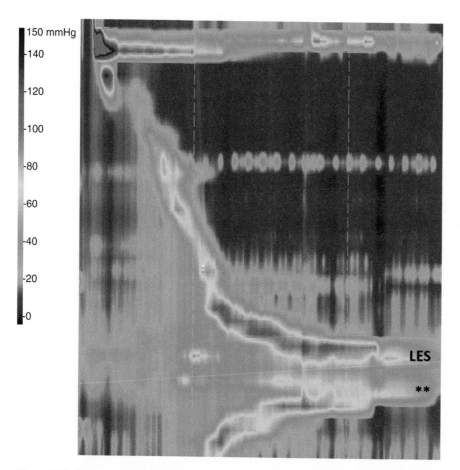

Figure 2.70 High-resolution esophageal manometry of folded manometry catheter. The LES pressure returns to baseline at the end of the wet swallow, but there is a "mirror-image" or "butterfly" pattern of the catheter just distal to the LES (*double asterisks*). To eliminate this artifact, the catheter should be pulled back and reinsertion attempted. A similar finding may also occur in patients with a large hiatal hernia or achalasia, in whom the catheter may not readily traverse the distal esophagus

Failed Impedance Sensors

Technical problems involving impedance sensors may be evident from sharp horizontal breaks that suggest improper recording (Fig. 2.72).

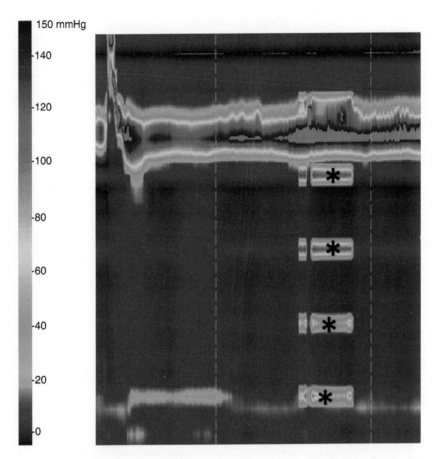

Figure 2.71 High-resolution esophageal manometry: Broken catheter sleeve. This catheter was malfunctioning; the pressure sensors are not correctly recording the circumferential pressures (*asterisks*). Initially, this type of malfunction may be intermittent, but ultimately complete malfunctioning of several sensors will require repair or replacement of the catheter

Failed Sensor Banks

Aberrant pressure recordings such as those seen in Figure 2.73 suggest that the cather requires repair or replacement.

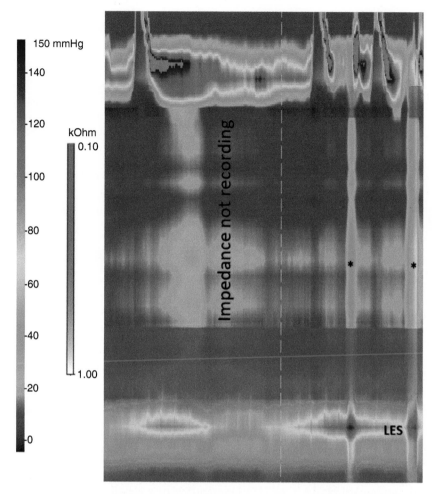

Figure 2.72 High-resolution esophageal manometry with impedance in achalasia type I: Failed impedance sensors. In this patient with achalasia type I, the bolus clearance is impeded by persistently elevated LES relaxation pressure and an absence of peristalsis, but there is clearly a technical issue with the impedance catheter's sensors proximal to the large purple area. The impedance plot shows a sharply marked horizontal line, which suggests that the more proximal impedance sensors are not recording properly. The *asterisks* demonstrate high-pressure columns originating from the gastric area, suggesting patient coughing during the data acquisition, preceded by a deep inspiration. There is no retrograde bolus movement or the UES does not relax; this is not emesis or retching

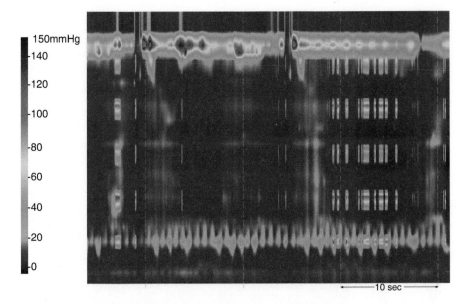

Figure 2.73 High-resolution esophageal manometry of failed sensor banks. The aberrant pressure recordings in this HRM are due to failed sensor banks. This catheter may need to be repaired or replaced, as it cannot measure esophageal pressure accurately

References

1. Kahrilas PJ, Bredenoord AJ, Fox M, Gyawali CP, Roman S, Smout AJ, Pandolfino JE, International High Resolution Manometry Working Group. The Chicago Classification of esophageal motility disorders, v3.0. Neurogastroenterol Motil. 2015;27:160–74.
2. Tutuian R, Castell DO. Clarification of the esophageal function defect in patients with manometric ineffective esophageal motility: studies using combined impedance-manometry. Clin Gastroenterol Hepatol. 2004;2:230–6.
3. Hiestand M, Abdel Jalil A, Castell DO. Manometric subtypes of ineffective esophageal motility. Clin Transl Gastroenterol. 2017;8:e78.
4. Ravi K, Murray JA, Geno DM, Katzka DA. Achalasia and chronic opiate use: innocent bystanders or associated conditions? Dis Esophagus. 2016;29:15–21.
5. Xiao Y, Kahrilas PJ, Kwasny MJ, Roman S, Lin Z, Nicodeme F, et al. High-resolution manometry correlates of ineffective esophageal motility. Am J Gastroenterol. 2012;107:1647–54.
6. Min YW, Shin I, Son HJ, Rhee PL. Multiple rapid swallow maneuver enhances the clinical utility of high-resolution manometry in patients showing ineffective esophageal motility. Medicine (Baltimore). 2015;94:e1669.
7. Vakil N, van Zanten SV, Kahrilas P, Dent J, Jones R, Global Consensus Group. The Montreal definition and classification of gastroesophageal reflux disease: a global evidence-based consensus. Am J Gastroenterol. 2006;101:1900–20.
8. Kimmel JN, Carlson DA, Hinchcliff M, Carns MA, Aren KA, Lee J, Pandolfino JE. The association between systemic sclerosis disease manifestations and esophageal high-resolution manometry parameters. Neurogastroenterol Motil. 2016;28:1157–65.
9. Halland M, Pandolfino J, Barba E. Diagnosis and treatment of rumination syndrome. Clin Gastroenterol Hepatol. 2018;16:1549–55.

Chapter 3
Antroduodenal Manometry

Overview

Gastric and small bowel motor activity is less commonly evaluated. Such evaluations usually are conducted only at expert centers, because of a number of factors. The first is that the placement of manometry catheters into the small bowel requires either fluoroscopic or endoscopic guidance. As a word of caution, the delicate nature of modern high-resolution manometry catheters makes them highly susceptible to damage. Endoscopic placement can be quite traumatic to the solid-state sensors, leading to expensive repair. Secondly, the data acquisition is time-consuming and labor-intensive. The final factor is the greater expertise required for the interpretation of these studies, which are more complex than esophageal studies and have not been the subject of extensive literature.

Antroduodenal manometry (ADM) allows for evaluation of the gastric, duodenal, and proximal jejunal motor function. Typically, the manometry catheter is placed across the gastric pyloric channel. Extending into at least the proximal 20 cm of the small bowel allows simultaneous pressure measurements of both the antrum and the duodenum. Owing to the challenges of this measurement, few studies have assessed this technique in disease states. This chapter concentrates on normal ADM during fasting and post-prandial periods, as well as appropriate response to intravenous promotility agents (e.g., erythromycin) for provocative testing.

ADM can be an important test in certain disease conditions, such as gastroparesis, myogenic and neurogenic chronic intestinal pseudo-obstruction (CIPO), and subacute partial small bowel obstruction; these are discussed in detail. Manometry is often the best method for the assessment of these conditions, which can be missed on routine radiographic evaluation.

© Springer Nature Switzerland AG 2020   95
S. Moosavi et al., *Atlas of High-Resolution Manometry, Impedance, and pH Monitoring*, https://doi.org/10.1007/978-3-030-27241-8_3

Indications

ADM can be considered as part of the workup for patients who have recurrent moderate to severe nausea, vomiting, abdominal pain, or bloating and distension without any intraluminal pathology on endoscopy and/or imaging. Patients who have gastroparesis on a gastric emptying study but fail to respond to initial therapy can be further evaluated by ADM to rule out small bowel dysmotility contributing to delayed gastric emptying. A common finding in patients with these symptoms is subacute partial small bowel obstruction, which can be missed on abdominal CT scans. In this instance, ADM detects a classic pattern of stationary, nonmigratory bursts of prolonged contractions (>30 minutes) [1]. ADM can also differentiate between neurogenic and myogenic chronic intestinal pseudo-obstruction; this distinction in some instances can guide therapy. Finally, in patients with severe constipation and colonic inertia who are being considered for colectomy, ADM can be used to assess the extent of bowel dysmotility. Although published data are limited, it is believed that patients with colonic inertia who have concomitant small bowel dysmotility may have a more guarded prognosis after colectomy, information that may help guide the patient's expectations.

Technique and Protocol

Generally, ADM catheters are inserted using fluoroscopic guidance. Therefore, to minimize the risk of intraprocedural aspiration, the patient is asked to fast for 8 hours before the procedure. In addition, migrating motor complexes (MMCs), the housekeeping waves that sweep the bowel of any residual debris, occur approximately every 90 minutes during fasting. Patients are instructed to withhold any medications that may impact gastric and small bowel motility, including anticholinergic medications and opioids.

A solid-state high-resolution manometry catheter is preferred for ADM even though it is more difficult to insert because of its less flexible material. The catheter is the same as the type used for esophageal manometry, incorporating 36 pressure sensors spaced at 1-cm intervals. After application of 2% lidocaine into the nostrils, the catheter is placed transnasally into the stomach under fluoroscopic guidance, usually without upper endoscopy. Subsequently, the catheter is advanced so that it crosses the antrum, extending into at least 20 cm of proximal small bowel. Patients do not receive systemic sedation, as studies have shown that medications such as midazolam increase the motility index of phase III, with longer duration, frequency, and contraction amplitudes of MMC III in the proximal and distal duodenum, and shorter MMC duration [2].

The patient then undergoes recording for a minimum of 4 hours while still fasting. This is followed by 1 hour of post-prandial recording. Provocative testing using medications such as IV erythromycin 50 mg is often performed just prior to meal ingestion to assess gastric and small bowel response. Erythromycin, a motilin receptor agonist, initiates a prolonged period of phasic gastric contractions and small bowel MMCs. During the study, the patient is asked to report any GI symptoms, including nausea, vomiting, or abdominal pain, to correlate the symptoms with manometric findings. It is recommended that diabetic patients have capillary blood glucose measurement before ADM, as hyperglycemia (plasma glucose level >15 mmol/L) is related to decreased antral motility and increased duodenal MMC cycle frequency because of significantly shorter phase II MMCs [3].

Normal ADM

In general, there are at least three phases of interdigestive (fasting) activity during ADM, termed the *fasting state motility pattern*—phase I, phase II, and phase III. The other state is termed the *fed state*. During the fasting period, the stomach is generally in a state of electromechanical dissociation. The gastric pacemaker is located between the proximal third of the stomach and the distal two thirds. The electrical activation is noted at a rate of 3 discharges per minute during electrogastrography, but in the fasting state, energy conservation prevents the stomach from responding to these frequent discharges. Even during fasting, however, infrequent low-amplitude contractions are seen.

Similar to the stomach, the small bowel has intrinsic pacesetter activity, but at a frequency of 11 cycles per minute. The small bowel too is mostly electromechanically dissociated during fasting. Only a pressure contraction greater than 10 mm Hg is considered significant [4].

Some terminology oddities in ADM need to be dealt with here. The first involves the term called the *migrating motor complex (MMC)*. Technically, the full MMC event represents the entire set of cycling from phase I through phase III, but convention has frequently misused the term to mean only phase III. This difference needs to be considered when reading the literature.

The three major distinct phases of fasting motility (of the MMC) are examined for their presence, propagation, and duration. Phase III is the most dynamic of the three events, and most texts start with describing phase III. During phase III of MMC, gastric antral contractions are the first to occur and are completely engaged at a frequency of three cycles per minute, often with amplitude >40 mm Hg. This is followed in sequence by a fully engaged duodenum with contractions at a frequency of 11 cycles per minute (Fig. 3.1). This phase III is a "migrating event"; it lasts for only a few minutes in any one location as it begins to travel from proximal to distal and projects down beyond the catheter. The way this event traverses is the reason phase III is interchangeably called the "migrating" motor complex (MMC), given such dramatic migration. The phase III MMC normally lasts about 3–4 minutes [5].

Once the phase III contraction passes distal to a sensor location, the bowel segment enters phase I, which is a period of quiescence (Fig. 3.2). Some believe that this occurs because the neuromuscular apparatus enters a refractory phase. Phase I

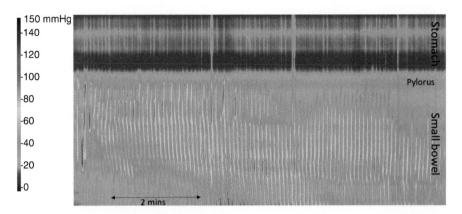

Figure 3.1   High-resolution antroduodenal manometry of a normal phase III MMC contraction during the fasting period. This phase lasted roughly 9 minutes. Phase III migrating motor complex (MMC) contractions generally start in the proximal duodenum, and sometimes in the gastric antrum. The fasting MMC duodenal contractions occur at a frequency of 11–12 cycles per minute. There is a normal antegrade propagation of these contractions. Each contraction is much easier to appreciate on the high-resolution tracing.

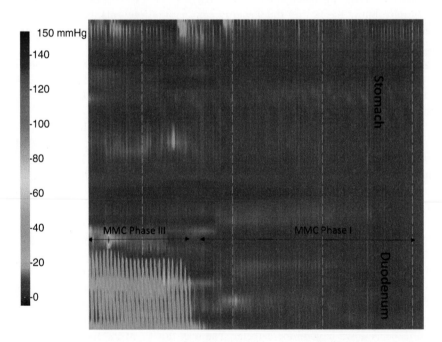

Figure 3.2   High-resolution antroduodenal manometry during the fasting period. There are frequent contractions (frequency, 11 cycles per minute) in the proximal duodenum. These are characteristic of MMC phase III, propagating antegrade along the small bowel. This phase lasts about 4–5 minutes, followed by the quiescent phase characteristic of phase I, which lasts approximately 50 minutes.

generally lasts for 40–50 minutes. Subsequently, phase II begins, which is characterized by irregular propagated contractions and some non-propagated contractions. During phase II, these events proceed with increasing frequency over time. They are typically more frequent, but with maximum rate less than slow wave frequency occurs (3 cycles per minute for gastric and 11 cycles per minute for duodenal segment) [6]. Phase II then culminates in phase III (Fig. 3.3). The total duration of the MMCs is typically 90–100 minutes during a fasting wake period [4]. Of note, occasionally a normal MMC originates from the duodenum, and not from the stomach.

The MMC is an important event. Another term used for this pattern during fasting is the "housekeeping wave," because the purpose of the MMC (particularly phase III) is to cleanse debris from the stomach and small bowel. The stomach and small bowel are vital for digestion, so (like a dirty plate) they need to be cleansed of non-digestible materials so these residues will not interfere with subsequent meal digestion and absorption. The lack of MMC has been implicated in the development of small intestinal bacterial overgrowth, suggesting that MMC also has a role in cleaning microbial buildup from this important part of the gut.

Eating completely changes the motor function of the proximal gut. Food ingestion immediately leads to cessation of MMCs, and the gut progresses to the "fed state." During ADMs, centers often use a standardized meal, such as Ensure (250 Kcal) to study a fed response during ADM. The amount of ingested meal should be recorded. The fed period ends when the phase III MMC returns, which usually occurs at least 2 hours after meal ingestion.

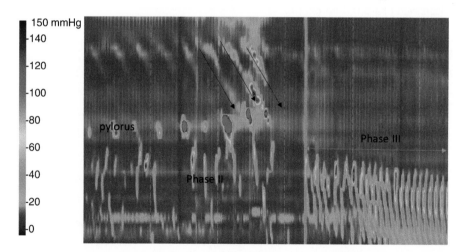

Figure 3.3 High-resolution antroduodenal manometry of a normal subject during the fasting period. Initially, this tracing shows irregular contractions in the proximal small bowel. Background gastric contractions at the frequency of 3 cycles per minute are seen in mid-stomach (*solid arrow*). There are phase II irregular contractions in the proximal small bowel. These are subsequently converted to phase III MMC regular contractions at the frequency of 11 cycles per minute; which propagate normally antegrade.

During the postprandial phase, high-amplitude, irregular contractions are seen in the gastric antrum, as the stomach grinds and mixes the solid food (Fig. 3.4). Lower amplitude, irregular contractions are seen in the duodenum with the presence of nutrients in the lumen (Fig. 3.5). The duration of this phase depends on the food content, consistency, and calories [4]. It is believed that duodeno-gastric coordination determines the timing and degree of gastric contraction for triturition and delivery of chyme to the small bowel, preparing to handle the next bolus. This coordination prevents food from simply being dumped into the duodenum.

Provocative testing during ADM can be important. It is particularly important when the ADM is abnormal. For example, if no phase III is seen, triggering a phase II with intravenous erythromycin can suggest that the problem is more neuropathic than myopathic. In myopathic conditions, nothing should provide a good response. Typically, IV erythromycin in healthy subjects produces longer and more vigorous phasic antral contractions, and a typical phase III lasting up to 15 minutes (Fig. 3.6). Usually, erythromycin induces phase III events of greater amplitude and duration. Sometimes, multiple phase III events are produced. The phase III contractions in the proximal duodenum show no difference in duration and frequency from spontaneously occurring phase III. After IV erythromycin, phase III in the proximal jejunum is shorter and has slower migration [7]. On the other hand, octreotide initiates small intestinal phase III activity but suppresses antral phase II activity during fasting and the post-prandial period in healthy subjects within 30 minutes of subcutaneous injection [8]. These increased MMC phase III activities have longer duration and greater propagation velocity than spontaneous MMCs and are associated with decreased phase II duration [9].

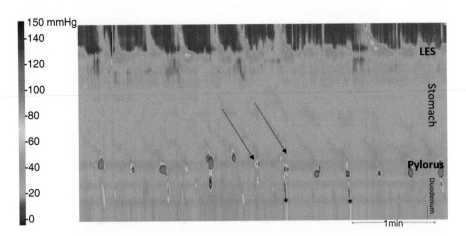

Figure 3.4 High-resolution antroduodenal manometry showing normal conversion from fasting to a "fed" pattern. Increased activity is seen in the stomach, with contractions of higher pressure amplitude with a frequency of three cycles per minute (*arrow*). There is intermittent duodenal acitivity (*asterisk*) without clusters, which is normal. The pylorus is contracting intermittently, which is physiologically normal as the stomach processes the food. LES—lower esophageal sphincter

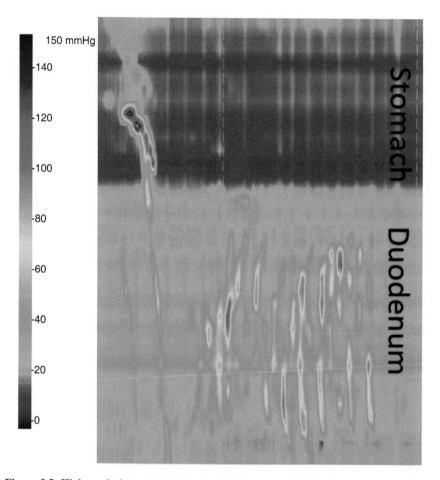

Figure 3.5 High-resolution antroduodenal manometry of MMC-III like (i.e., cluster) contractions in proximal small bowel during the fed state. During the fed state, the antrum contracts, while the proximal small bowel remains quiescent unless there is nutrient in proximal duodenum, which leads to intermittent contractions of the duodenum and proximal jejunum. Therefore, it is abnormal to see clusters of contractions in the proximal small bowel during the fed phase; they may be suggestive of neurogenic dysmotility. In this figure, there are no significant repetitive antral contractions, a state that may take 20 minutes after the onset of the meal to appear.

Abnormal ADM Pattern

There are various patterns to look for when considering ADM as part of a diagnostic approach. If the patterns indicated above are all present, the manometry is considered to be normal. However, there are features that need to be considered.

One of the most common findings during manometry is a diminished intensity or frequency of MMC cycling. The absence of phase III is characteristic of this pattern. When this pattern is seen, there are several considerations. Opiates can reduce the frequency of MMCs, and studies have shown that anticholinergic medication such as neo-

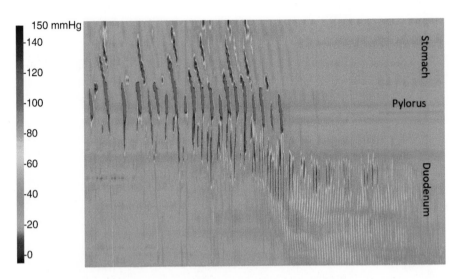

Figure 3.6 High-resolution antroduodenal manometry of MMC-like contractions after 50 mg IV erythromycin. Erythromycin is a motilin agonist that promotes motility. These contractions are initiated in the stomach and are propagated into the small bowel, a normal response to erythromycin. This pattern may be absent in patients with myopathic chronic intestinal pseudo-obstruction.

stigmine can increase antral and intestinal motor activity in patients with hypomotility [10]. However, the lack of MMC can also be seen in irritable bowel syndrome (IBS) and small intestinal bacterial overgrowth and usually represents a form of neuropathy of the gut [10]. In addition, exogenous glucagon-like peptide 1 (GLP-1) agonists have shown to slow gastric emptying in healthy, obese, and type II diabetic subjects [11–13]. Therefore, the patient's medication history should be reviewed before ADM.

Patients with intestinal pseudo-obstruction associated with enteric neuropathy generally have a preserved but uncoordinated pattern or propagation of MMC or MMC phase III contractions. In autonomic (extrinsic) neuropathy, impaired fed response with postprandial antral hypomobility is observed [14]. Other patterns that may be seen with neuropathic variation include bursts of non-propagated phasic pressure activity (duration >20 minutes, amplitude >20 mm Hg, frequency >10 waves/minute) during the fasting period and/or a fed state, with sustained, uncoordinated fasting pressure activity (duration >30 minutes). These bursts are called *cluster contractions* (i.e., MMC phase III–like contractions) [15] (Fig. 3.7). Another sign of neuropathy is the inability to convert from the fasting pattern to the fed pattern after an ingested meal. For example, seeing a phase III in the post-prandial state is quite abnormal. In type 1 diabetes or long-standing type 2 diabetes, most patients have autonomic neuropathy, which can be evident from an infrequent antral component of MMC and decreased antral contraction during the post-prandial period, with normal amplitude or antral hypomotility [16].

In chronic myogenic intestinal pseudo-obstruction, MMCs can be preserved, but with very low-amplitude contractions, generally less than 20 mm Hg [14] (Fig. 3.8). The stomach contractions can be preserved during the early stage, but in the late stage of severe visceral myopathy, the normal MMC pattern is absent or cannot be identified because of the very low amplitude of contractions. This pattern can be

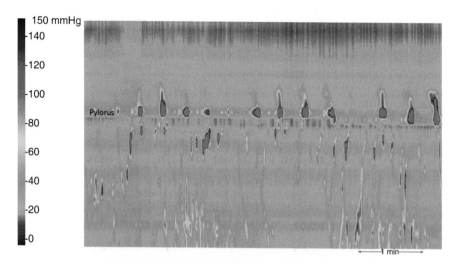

Figure 3.7 High-resolution antroduodenal manometry of a patient with a neurogenic variant of chronic intestinal pseudo-obstruction during the fasting period. There are clusters of MMC-like contractions in the proximal small bowel during the meal phase. These clusters of contractions are non-propagating. There are also high-pressure contractions in the pylorus, which are not normal.

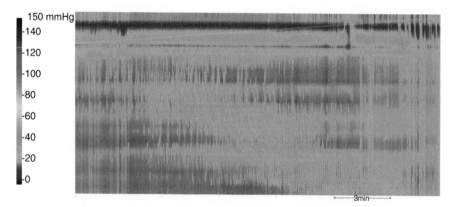

Figure 3.8 High-resolution antroduodenal manometry of a patient with myogenic variant of chronic intestinal pseudo-obstruction during the fasting period. In this HRM, there are low-amplitude, MMC-like contractions during the fasting state.

seen in patients with systemic sclerosis, amyloidosis, muscular dystrophy, and familial myopathic CIPO. In fact, in the extreme stage of these conditions, little or no motor activity is detectable.

Another potential use of ADM is the detection of partial small bowel obstruction, which can have a very distinctive motor pattern. This test can then be important when abdominal imaging may not identify the small bowel obstruction in patients with recurrent nausea, vomiting, and decreased oral tolerance. Therefore, ADM is indicated, as it can identify certain patterns more consistent with subacute low-grade small bowel obstruction. In mechanical obstruction, frequent non-propagated and prolonged contraction, cluster of contractions, or bursts of rhythmic phasic activity lasting for more than 30 minutes can be seen on high-resolution ADM (Fig. 3.9). Retrograde contractions may also be seen (Fig. 3.10). Patients should be referred for exploratory laparotomy to further assess the underlying etiology of the small bowel obstruction [1, 17].

Other abnormal patterns on ADM can show pylorospasm (Fig. 3.11), folded catheters (Figs. 3.12 and 3.13), or gastroparesis (Fig. 3.14).

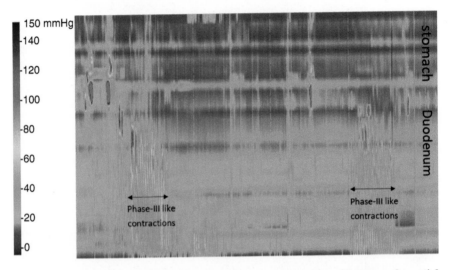

Figure 3.9 High-resolution antroduodenal manometry of a patient with low-grade partial small bowel obstruction. There are repetitive, simultaneous, non-propagating phase III–like contractions. There is no phase I quiescent period, which is normally about 40–50 minutes in duration. This pattern is suggestive of subacute partial small bowel obstruction.

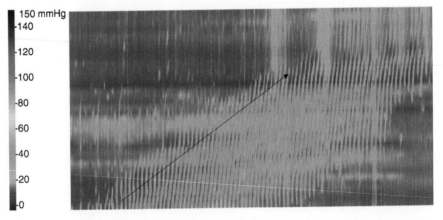

Figure 3.10 High-resolution antroduodenal manometry of retrograde small bowel contractions in a patient with Roux-en-Y gastric bypass surgery. The patient presented with recurrent nausea, vomiting, decreased oral intake, and weight loss. The upper endoscopy and imaging were unremarkable. The ADM shows retrograde contraction in the small bowel. The exploratory laparotomy identified a reversed anastomosis at the Y-limb.

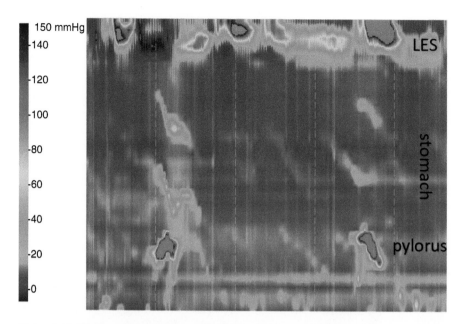

Figure 3.11 High-resolution antroduodenal manometry of hypercontractile pressure in the pylorus. The contraction amplitude is 360 mm Hg. There is no updated definition for the criteria of pylorospasm on high-resolution solid-state ADM; previous definitions in the literature have suggested that patients with pylorospasm exhibit pyloric contraction >10 mm Hg and longer than 3 minutes in duration. In this study, the background contraction of the pylorus was roughly 10 mm Hg, so the overall pattern is highly suggestive of pylorospasm. Baseline gastric contractions are observed at a rate of three per minute.

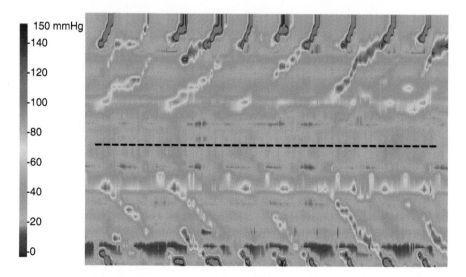

Figure 3.12 High-resolution antroduodenal manometry post-emesis. After the patient vomited during the study, the catheter was dislodged from its original position and folded in the stomach. The gastric contraction patterns are mirror-image across the dotted line; this "butterfly" effect is compatible with a folded catheter.

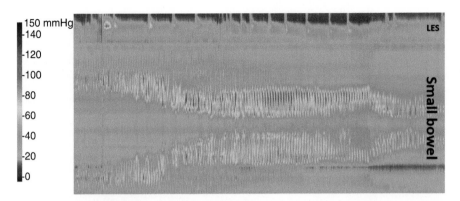

Figure 3.13 High-resolution antroduodenal manometry of a folded catheter in the small bowel in a patient with gastrectomy. A mirror-image pattern indicates a folded catheter. Note the distal esophageal contraction proximal to the LES. There are also phase III MMC-like contractions initiated from the proximal small bowel and propagating antegrade.

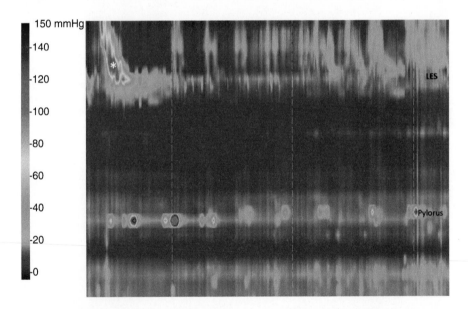

Figure 3.14 High-resolution antroduodenal manometry after a standard meal intake in a patient with gastroparesis. With conversion to a post-prandial pattern, normally the gastric contractile activities increase and the small bowel contractions decrease. In this study, no appropriate post-prandial pattern is seen. There is no gastric activity here, with intermittent and infrequent low-amplitude contractions in the pylorus. These findings are suggestive of gastroparesis. Note the distal esophageal peristalsis above the LES.

In summary, high-resolution ADM offers further insight into the gastric and small bowel motor physiology, offering greater clarity than conventional tracings. In the right hands, the interpretation of abnormal foregut motor patterns can help to identify some conditions and may even determine the potential benefits of various therapies.

References

1. Frank JW, Sarr MG, Camilleri M. Use of gastroduodenal manometry to differentiate mechanical and functional intestinal obstruction: an analysis of clinical outcome. Am J Gastroenterol. 1994;89:339–44.
2. Castedal M, Björnsson E, Abrahamsson H. Effects of midazolam on small bowel motility in humans. Aliment Pharmacol Ther. 2000;14:571–7.
3. Gielkens HA, Verkijk M, Frölich M, Lamers CB, Masclee AA. Is the effect of acute hyperglycaemia on interdigestive antroduodenal motility and small-bowel transit mediated by insulin? Eur J Clin Invest. 1997;27:703–10.
4. Bortolotti M, Annese V, Coccia G. Twenty-four hour ambulatory antroduodenal manometry in normal subjects (co-operative study). Neurogastroenterol Motil. 2000;12:231–8.
5. Kellow JE, Borody TJ, Phillips SF, Tucker RL, Haddad AC. Human interdigestive motility: variations in patterns from esophagus to colon. Gastroenterology. 1986;91:386–95.
6. Holland R, Gallagher MD, Quigley EM. An evaluation of an ambulatory manometry system in assessment of antroduodenal motor activity. Dig Dis Sci. 1996;41:1531–7.
7. Björnsson ES, Abrahamsson H. Comparison between physiologic and erythromycin-induced interdigestive motility. Scand J Gastroenterol. 1995;30:139–45.
8. Chen JD, Lin ZY, Edmunds MC, McCallum RW. Effects of octreotide and erythromycin on gastric myoelectrical and motor activities in patients with gastroparesis. Dig Dis Sci. 1998;43:80–9.
9. Haruma K, Wiste JA, Camilleri M. Effect of octreotide on gastrointestinal pressure profiles in health and in functional and organic gastrointestinal disorders. Gut. 1994;35:1064–9.
10. Parthasarathy G, Ravi K, Camilleri M, Andrews C, Szarka LA, Low PA, et al. Effect of neostigmine on gastroduodenal motility in patients with suspected gastrointestinal motility disorders. Neurogastroenterol Motil. 2015;27:1736–46.
11. Little TJ, Pilichiewicz AN, Russo A, Phillips L, Jones KL, Nauck MA, et al. Effects of intravenous glucagon-like peptide-1 on gastric emptying and intragastric distribution in healthy subjects: relationships with postprandial glycemic and insulinemic responses. J Clin Endocrinol Metab. 2006;91:1916–23.
12. Näslund E, Gutniak M, Skogar S, Rössner S, Hellström PM. Glucagon-like peptide 1 increases the period of postprandial satiety and slows gastric emptying in obese men. Am J Clin Nutr. 1998;68:525–30.
13. Meier JJ, Gallwitz B, Salmen S, Goetze O, Holst JJ, Schmidt WE, Nauck MA. Normalization of glucose concentrations and deceleration of gastric emptying after solid meals during intravenous glucagon-like peptide 1 in patients with type 2 diabetes. J Clin Endocrinol Metab. 2003;88:2719–25.
14. Bharucha AE, Camilleri M, Low PA, Zinsmeister AR. Autonomic dysfunction in gastrointestinal motility disorders. Gut. 1993;34:397–401.
15. Verhagen MA, Samsom M, Jebbink RJ, Smout AJ. Clinical relevance of antroduodenal manometry. Eur J Gastroenterol Hepatol. 1999;11:523–8.
16. Samsom M, Jebbink RJ, Akkermans LM, Berge-Henegouwen GP, Smout AJ. Abnormalities of antroduodenal motility in type I diabetes. Diabetes Care. 1996;19:21–7.
17. Patcharatrakul T, Gonlachanvit S. Technique of functional and motility test: how to perform antroduodenal manometry. J Neurogastroenterol Motil. 2013;19:395–404.

Chapter 4
Anorectal Manometry

Overview

High-resolution anorectal manometry is a technique that allows dynamic assessment of pelvic floor muscles, particularly the puborectalis muscle of the levator ani complex and the internal and external anal sphincters. These muscles are assessed both during rest and during certain maneuvers. The principle of anorectal manometry is similar to that of the esophageal manometry.

The advantages of high-resolution anorectal manometry compared with the conventional (water-perfused) technique may not be as pronounced as the advantages of esophageal or antroduodenal manometry. Given the short length of the anal canal, it is feasible to have more sensors closely spaced along the conventional catheter. According to a recent study by Lee et al. [1], there is a good correlation between conventional and high-resolution anorectal manometry. The high-resolution anorectal catheter is thought to be better, however, for assessing the anal sphincter length and pressures during the bear down maneuver on the commode. In addition, the two techniques are poorly correlated in subtypes of dyssynergic defecation. With higher resolution, more pressure details can be seen along the anal pressure segments. The color-pressure contour follows the same principle as in esophageal high-resolution manometry, with cool colors representing lower pressure and warm colors for high pressures.

The high-resolution catheter has multiple pressure sensors that allow simultaneous assessment of anorectal pressures. Two types of high-resolution anorectal manometry catheters are available:

- *Three-dimensional high-definition anorectal manometry (HDARM):* This solid-state rigid catheter (Medtronic® ManoScan™) is 10.75 mm in diameter and has 256 pressure points, generated by 16 axial and 16 circumferential sensors. The spacing between circumferential sensors is 2 mm; axial sensors are 4 mm apart. The length of the catheter is 64 mm. This catheter is capable of recording pressure points radially and longitudinally. An inflatable detachable balloon is

S. Moosavi et al., *Atlas of High-Resolution Manometry, Impedance, and pH Monitoring*, https://doi.org/10.1007/978-3-030-27241-8_4

Figure 4.1 High-resolution anorectal manometry catheter with and without the rectal balloon. The catheter has 256 pressure sensors. The deflated balloon is mounted upon the tip of the catheter. The catheter with the mounted balloon is inserted into the rectum

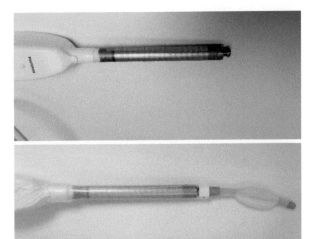

mounted on the proximal end of the catheter. The balloon can be inflated to various pressures, allowing the assessment of the rectoanal inhibitory reflex and rectal sensations.

- *High-resolution anorectal manometry catheter (HRARM):* This solid-state flexible catheter (Medtronic®) is 4.2 mm in diameter and consists of 10 circumferential copper pressure sensors at 6-mm intervals along its shaft, with two additional pressure sensors at the proximal tip of the catheter (Fig. 4.1). This catheter is only capable of recording longitudinal pressure points. Medical Measurement Systems and Sandhill Scientific also offer HRARM catheters with similar constructs.

As with high-resolution esophageal manometry catheters, pressure measurements by anorectal manometry catheters drift with changes in temperature (thermal drift). Hence, thermal compensation is required at the time of data analysis, but because the procedure time for anorectal manometry is less than for esophageal or antroduodenal manometry, the degree of thermal drift is less prominent.

Technique

To accurately evaluate the anorectal function, the patient ideally evacuates the rectum, spontaneously or by using an enema, 2–3 hours before the procedure. Patients can carry on their normal activities of daily living before the procedure, including eating, drinking, and taking routine medications. However, the medications list should be obtained before the procedure, as medications could contribute to some symptoms, including diarrhea or constipation.

The details of the procedure should be discussed thoroughly with the patient before the study, especially the various maneuvers that will be done during the study. The patient should be coached to remain calm and relaxed during the study, as an anxious patient may contract the abdominal muscles or external anal sphincters, which could affect the pressure measurements on manometry. In addition, it is crucial that the patient has the communication skills and the mental capacity to understand and follow various maneuvers requested during the procedure.

Before initiating the study, follow the manufacturer's instructions to calibrate the catheter to "zero" to atmospheric level and "maximum or high-point" calibration. Further details of calibration should be reviewed with the manufacturer. The inflatable balloon is attached to the proximal end of the catheter. Lubricant on a cotton gauze is required to perform the digital rectal exam and to facilitate the insertion of the anorectal manometry catheter and attached balloon into the rectum. When using the HDARM catheter, it is important to place the catheter with the appropriate orientation in the rectum, with the aspect marked "posterior" positioned towards the coccyx. This positioning allows evaluation of a sphincter defect or any other abnormalities in an anatomically correct position. The most distal sensor of the catheter should be placed a centimeter caudally from the anus.

Protocol

After explaining the details of the evaluation to the patient, the study is started by performing a comprehensive digital rectal exam in the left lateral decubitus position. The complete details of this exam are beyond the scope of this book. Briefly, the anus and perineum are visualized for any skin rash or lesion, while the patient remains in the left lateral decubitus position throughout the study. The anus is exposed to visualize any fissures, perianal fistulae, skin tags, hemorrhoids, or condylomata. The patient is asked to "squeeze" and "bear down" to visualize the sphincters and perineal movements. The anocutaneous reflex is assessed with a cotton swab, which allows testing of the integrity of the S2, S3, and S4 nerve roots by stroking the perianal skin in four quadrants towards the anus, where intact motor neurons lead to contraction of the anal sphincter. A lubricated, gloved finger is then slowly inserted in the rectum to assess for mass, stricture, and tenderness. The pulp of the index finger should face posteriorly, with the anal sphincter at the level of the proximal interphalangeal joint. This position allows for better perception of anal sphincter contraction and relaxation. Contraction of the puborectalis muscle can be perceived on the distal interphalangeal joint of the index finger. The examiner should also evaluate the rectal vault for any impacted stool and its consistency. The sphincter tone, its length, and the anorectal angle are assessed at rest. The subject is then asked to "squeeze the finger" or "hold the stool," which assesses the squeeze pressure of the sphincters. In a normal response, the examiner's finger is pulled antero-superiorly by the puborectalis and external sphincter contractions. The exam is followed by a push effort during simulated defecation or "bear down." The opposite hand should be placed on the abdomen, to assess whether the patient is able to generate adequate intra-abdominal pressure required during defecation.

A normal response during defecation is abdominal muscle contraction, relaxation of anal sphincters and puborectalis muscles, and perineal descent of less than 4 centimeters [2].

Subsequently, the anorectal manometry catheter with the mounted balloon is lubricated and gently inserted into the rectum. Similar to the digital rectal exam, the patient should be placed in the left lateral decubitus position with hips and knees flexed to an angle of >90 degrees. If there is any pain, the insertion should be stopped, and the probe should be pulled back. Insertion can be attempted again, if the patient is agreeable. Once the probe is inserted, the patient is asked to remain quiet, with no voluntary contraction of abdominal muscles or anal sphincters. Generally, a "run-in" period of 3–5 minutes is allotted to allow the patient to get accustomed to the probe in the rectum before the study is recorded for the resting pressure measurement [3]. The resting pressure is measured for 1 minute. This allows detailed evaluation of the internal anal sphincter, which is responsible for 70% of continence at rest. In addition, the HDARM allows the visualization of the puborectalis muscle contraction, which contributes to the anorectal angle and the "flap-valve" mechanism of continence.

The patient is then asked to do a series of maneuvers, starting with a "squeeze" or "holding on to stool" for as long as possible, with a maximum of 30 seconds. This is usually repeated once more, with 30 seconds rest in between. The "squeeze" maneuver assesses the volitional effort of the anal sphincter pressure, predominantly from the external anal sphincter and puborectalis muscles. Following 30 seconds of rest, the patient is then asked to simulate evacuation. This maneuver examines the coordinated relaxation of the rectal and anal sphincters with appropriate rise in intra-rectal pressure (i.e., abdominal wall muscle contraction). In selected patients with fecal incontinence, a "cough reflex" may be tested to assess whether the anal sphincter pressure appropriately increases during an abrupt rise in intra-abdominal pressure with coughing. This maneuver may be repeated once.

Following the above maneuvers, the rectal sensation and rectoanal inhibitory reflex (RAIR) are evaluated with sequential balloon inflation and deflation, to a progressively larger volume of air. Thresholds of the first sensation, first urge to defecate, and severe urgency are recorded to evaluate rectal hyposensitivity or hypersensitivity. The balloon is first inflated to 20 mL, followed by deflation. The incremental increase in the balloon volume is usually 20 mL. The maximum inflated volume is 250 mL, as volumes larger than 250 mL do not provide any further valuable information to the evaluation. During the sequentially larger balloon inflations, there is a rapid relaxation of the internal anal sphincter by 25% or more from the basal pressure in response to the rapid inflation of the rectal balloon, followed by return to its baseline pressure once the balloon is deflated. This is referred to as RAIR (*see below* for details). The catheter is then removed, and the study is ended.

In patients who have anorectal manometric findings of dyssynergia or evacuation disorders, a balloon expulsion test ensues. A non-latex balloon is inserted in the rectum and is inflated with water to 50–60 mL. The patient is then asked to expel the balloon into a bedside commode. The ability to expel the balloon in less than 1 minute is considered normal [4].

Indications

Table 4.1 summarizes the various indication for high-resolution anorectal manometry. Patients with fecal incontinence or constipation may be referred for anorectal manometry, but the clinical history is extremely important in a thorough evaluation of these patients. Depending on the clinical history, patients may require endoscopic evaluation and other ancillary imaging, including pelvic imaging and MR or barium defecography.

For example, in patients with constipation, history of urgency, straining, and sensation of incomplete evacuation in the absence of endoscopic abnormality, with suboptimal response to laxatives or secretagogues, dyssynergic defecation should be considered. There may be evidence of paradoxical contraction of the anal sphincter muscles or lack of appropriate relaxation with simulated evacuation. Patients with dyssynergic defecation have symptoms of constipation with two out of three findings of abnormal, dyssynergic pattern of defecation on anorectal manometry, failed balloon expulsion test, and/or abnormal barium or MR defecography [5]. In addition, defecography is a useful diagnostic test in patients suspicious for rectocele, sigmoidocele, enterocele, rectal intussusception, rectal prolapse, and excessive perineal descent.

Dyssynergic defecation patterns may also occur in patients with ileal pouch anal anastomosis (IPAA) [6]. However, patients with a previous history of ulcerative colitis with IPAA pouch should undergo complete evaluation to rule out other etiologies, such as acute or chronic recurrent pouchitis, cuffitis, anal stricture, infectious colitis, ischemic pouchitis, or Crohn's disease, before referral to anorectal manometry.

Patients with fecal incontinence should be further questioned on the frequency, quantity, and consistency of fecal incontinence. It is pertinent to differentiate between seepage, urge, and passive incontinence. Urge incontinence may be due to rectal hypersensitivity and/or decreased rectal compliance. Passive incontinence is more likely to present with larger-volume fecal soiling and is likely to be due to diminished pressure of the external anal sphincters to provide voluntary continence with a progressive rise in rectal pressure and volume due to accumulated stool. Seepage generally occurs after a recent bowel movement and can occur in the setting

Table 4.1 Common indications for anorectal manometry and rectal sensitivity assessment	Chronic constipation, including defecatory disorders such as dyssynergic defecation
	Hirschsprung's disease
	Fecal incontinence (urge or passive)
	Functional anorectal pain
	Functional disorders of ileal pouch anal anastomosis (IPAA, J-pouch)
	Work-up of colonic reanastomosis to assess integrity of sphincter function
	Assessment before biofeedback therapy

of large internal hemorrhoids. These patients generally do not report gas incontinence, unlike those with urge or passive incontinence.

Patients with functional anal pain without anal fissures, anorectal mass, or other extraluminal pelvic pathologies can be assessed for rectal hypersensitivity or dyssynergic defecatory patterns, as biofeedback may provide symptomatic relief. Evaluation in this patient cohort often involves anoscopy, colonoscopy or flexible sigmoidoscopy and pelvic imaging to exclude alternative etiologies.

Finally, patients who are planned to undergo colonic reanastomosis surgery may benefit from anorectal manometry before surgical intervention, to assess the integrity of sphincter function.

Normal High-Resolution Anorectal Manometry

Anal Sphincter Functions

Fecal continence is normally maintained by various anatomical barriers, including pelvic floor muscles, internal and external anal sphincters, rectoanal angle (i.e., a "flap valve") created by the sling of puborectalis muscle, and rectoanal sensory innervations [7]. The internal anal sphincter (IAS) contributes to 70% of anal resting tone. The rest of this pressure is generated by the external anal sphincter (EAS), puborectalis muscle, and hemorrhoidal plexus. Normally, as stool accumulates in the rectum, the subject gradually develops a sensation of urgency. This is accompanied by reflex relaxation of the IAS and semi-voluntary relaxation of the pelvic floor muscles. The EAS contracts to provide continence until it is socially appropriate to defecate. The EAS then relaxes to allow passage of the stool in conjunction with Valsalva (i.e., abdominal wall muscle contractions) and an increase in intrarectal pressure, as well as the relaxation of the IAS.

The normal range of resting and squeeze pressures differs between males, nulliparous females, and parous females. In addition, the length of the anal sphincter differs in these groups. Because of the small sample size of anorectal manometry studies and the use of variable protocols, the exact normal range of resting and contractile pressures of anal sphincters is not yet unified.

Resting Anal Sphincter Pressure

Resting anal sphincter pressure is defined as the average maximum pressure (mm Hg) over the functional anal canal length during the 1-minute period of rest (Fig. 4.2). Functional anal canal length is the segment in which the pressure exceeds rectal pressure by 5 mm Hg or more. According to a study by Carrington et al. [8], normal mean resting anal sphincter pressure in women is 65 ± 19 mm Hg, with the minimum found to be 25 mm Hg and the maximum, 111 mm Hg. In men, the

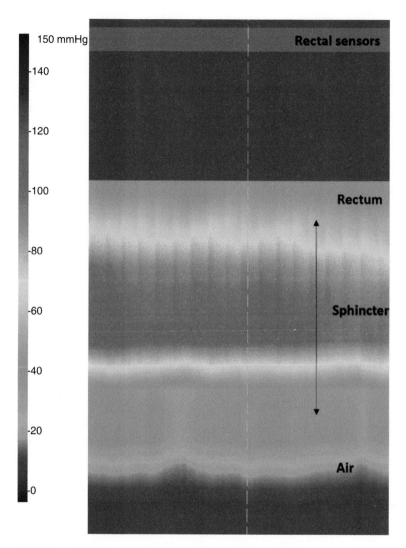

Figure 4.2 Normal high-resolution anorectal manometry at rest. With the patient lying in the left lateral decubitus position, the catheter is inserted into the anorectal cavity. The pressure is on the y-axis, and time is on the x-axis. The catheter's balloon sits in the rectum about 3 cm proximal to the most proximal sensor. At rest, there is a horizontal high-pressure zone in the anal canal, corresponding to the resting pressure generated by the puborectalis muscle and the anal sphincter. The most distal part of the illustration is the area outside of the subject (air). The normal resting anal pressure depends on sex and parity. Generally, normal mean resting anal sphincter pressure in women is 65 + 19 mmHg. In men, the normal mean resting anal sphincter is 73 + 23 mmHg. In this ARM, the mean absolute resting anal pressure is 94 mmHg

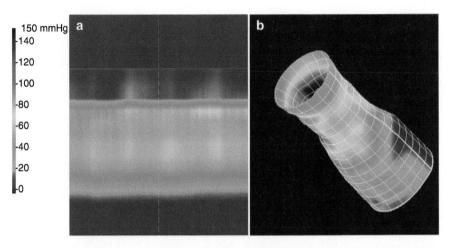

Figure 4.3 High-resolution anorectal manometry at rest. A, The resting pressure of the internal anal sphincter appears normal in this two-dimensional view. **B,** A three-dimensional view allows a better assessment of the integrity of the sphincter complex. Even though the overall complex appears normal on the two-dimensional view, one could appreciate that the sphincter complex does not generate equal pressure throughout its circumference. This is partly due to the resting pressure of the puborectalis muscle along the posterior anal canal, at the anorectal junction. There is no discernable sphincter defect. Therefore, this is a normal anorectal manometry at rest on both views

normal mean resting anal sphincter pressure is 73 ± 23 mm Hg, with a minimum of 38 mm Hg and a maximum of 136 mm Hg.

An increase in resting anal sphincter pressure can be seen in patients with anal fissure, anal pain, constipation, or anxiety during the test. These patients may also have ultra-slow waves at rest [9] (*See* Figure 4.16.) A lower resting anal sphincter pressure could be suggestive of IAS injury. Sphincter defects can be further evaluated with three-dimensional (3D)/2D images of high-resolution anorectal manometry (Fig. 4.3), as further discussed in a later section. Figures 4.4 and 4.5 illustrate other examples of resting anal sphincter pressure.

Anal Squeeze Pressure

The anal squeeze maneuver evaluates predominantly the EAS, which is a striated muscle and is under voluntary control. Intuitively, this pressure is lower in women than in men, and is lower in older patients than in younger ones. Therefore, it is stratified based on age and sex [10]. The maximum anal squeeze pressure range is quite different in various literature citations, but it is believed that the maximum absolute anal squeeze pressure ranges from 90 to 397 mm Hg in all females (86–387 mm Hg in parous females and 89–447 mm Hg in nulliparous females) and from 94 to 590 mm Hg in males [8]. Of note, the squeeze pressure also originates from contraction of the levator ani muscles, including the puborectalis muscle (Fig. 4.6).

Various alterations in squeeze pressure can be seen. For example, high squeeze pressure may be seen occasionally in men with chronic pelvic pain [10]. A weak

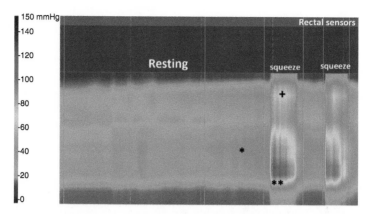

Figure 4.4 High-resolution anorectal manometry with diminished resting anal sphincter tone. The first approximately 30 seconds of this study is during the rest period. Initially, the anal sphincter pressure is relatively low, about 30 mm Hg. As time passes, the internal sphincter and puborectalis muscle slowly recover (*asterisk*), although the pressure remains within the low limit of normal. Therefore, it is advised to allot up to 3 minutes at the beginning of the study recording to allow the patient to get accustomed to having the catheter in place. The length of the functional anal sphincter is fairly short, about 2.5 cm in length. Note that the two squeeze maneuvers shown here are normal, with an appropriate rise in pressure to 100 mm Hg. The patient is recruiting the external anal sphincter (*double asterisks*) during the squeeze period. Also seen is a relative rise in pressure due to pelvic floor muscles (*plus sign*)

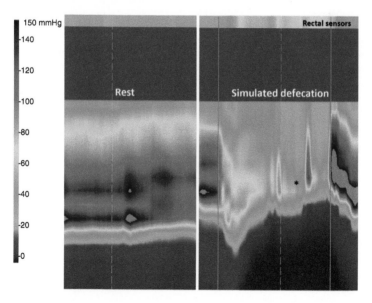

Figure 4.5 High-resolution anorectal manometry. A, Hypertensive resting anal sphincter. The pressure is 175 mm Hg. This finding may be seen in patients with constipation, anal fissure, or functional anal pain, but most often it results from the patient's anxiety during the evaluation. **B,** With an attempted defecation, the anal sphincters and puborectalis muscle relax appropriately, as seen by a drop in the pressure (*asterisk*). The patient appropriately recruits the abdominal muscle during the defecation, as seen by a rise in pressure along the rectal sensors. Given the artificial setting of the anorectal manometry, observation of a complete and perfect relaxation of the anal sphincter during manometry is rather rare

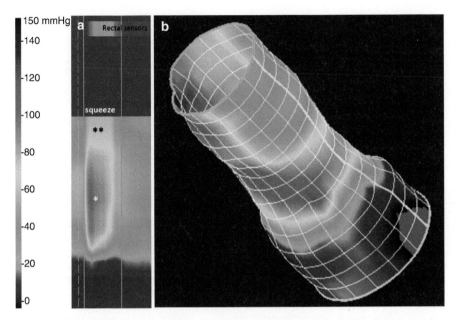

Figure 4.6 High-resolution anorectal manometry of a normal "squeeze" maneuver. A, Contraction of the puborectalis muscle and the external anal sphincter is seen as a high-pressure band (*asterisk*). In addition, the pelvic floor contracts with the "squeeze" maneuver (*double asterisks*), although this is less contributory. **B,** Three-dimensional view of a simulated squeeze maneuver allows differentiation of the asymmetrical area of high pressure generated by the contraction of the puborectalis muscle, which acts as a sling around the posterior aspect of the distal rectum, at the rectoanal junction. The rest of the circumferential high-pressure zone is likely due to the internal and external anal sphincters, as they contract during the squeeze maneuver

anal squeeze pressure may be due to an incomplete attempt by the patient. Therefore, if a weak squeeze is seen, the patient should be instructed to make maximum effort during the maneuver. Persistently low anal squeeze pressure could suggest weakness of the EAS and puborectalis muscles due to muscle or nerve injuries (such as a pudendal nerve injury). When interpreting the results, it is important to highlight both the absolute anal squeeze pressure and the relative change compared with the resting pressure (Fig. 4.7).

In addition, the duration of the anal squeeze is important. The EAS is a slow-twitch, fatigue-resistant type of striated muscle. A squeeze duration less than 10 seconds on non–high-resolution anorectal manometry has shown to be associated with impaired continence to liquid, but not solid stool [11].

Cough Reflex

In patients who have fecal incontinence, the EAS can be further assessed by asking them to cough or blow a balloon while the anal sphincter pressure is simultaneously measured. These maneuvers transiently increase intra-abdominal pressure. In a

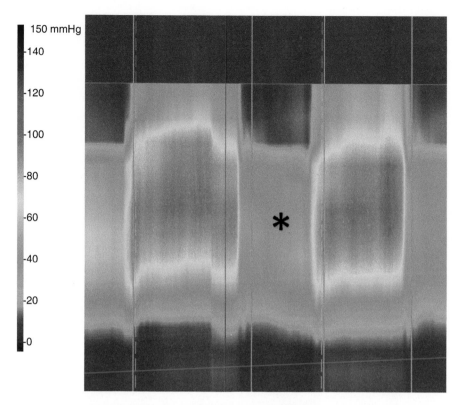

Figure 4.7 High-resolution anorectal manometry during simulated squeeze maneuver. Two-dimensional view of a simulated squeeze maneuver, demonstrating the normal contraction of the puborectalis muscle and the external anal sphincter. There is an increase in pressure compared with the baseline pressure (*asterisk*)

normal subject, such a rise in pressure leads to volitional EAS contraction to further enhance continence (Fig. 4.8). This reflex is mediated by the sacral reflex arc [12]. Low squeeze EAS pressure with a normal cough reflex could suggest impaired volitional control of the EAS or central spinal cord injury above the sacral area. On the other hand, if the patient has both low squeeze pressure and impaired cough reflex, then there is an injury to the sacral reflex arc.

Rectoanal Inhibitory Reflex (RAIR)

The RAIR is a local reflex through the myenteric plexus between the rectum and the anal canal. The exact role of this reflex is unknown, but it is postulated to serve as a "sampling reflex" of the rectal vault content, including gas, stool, or liquid [13]. In addition, it is an essential part of normal defecation. As the rectal volume increases with accumulating larger volume of stool, the internal anal sphincter progressively relaxes in preparation for defecation, if it is socially convenient. If so, the IAS, EAS,

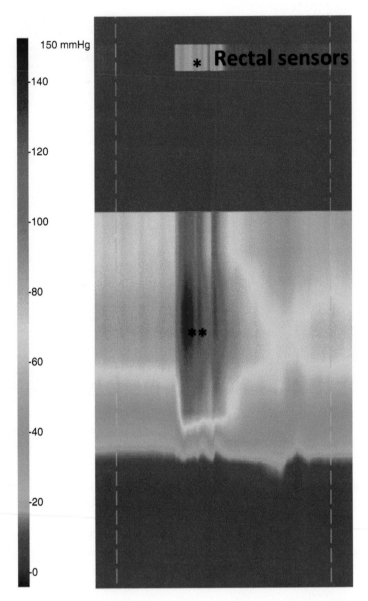

Figure 4.8 High-resolution anorectal manometry while the patient coughs. The intrarectal (i.e., intra-abdominal) pressure rises sharply during cough (*asterisk*). The cough initiates a sacral reflex causing contraction of the external anal sphincter and puborectalis muscle, shown as a rapid increase in pressure (*double asterisks*). The pressure returns to baseline after the cough. Patients with sacral nerve root or pudendal nerve injuries do not have this reflex

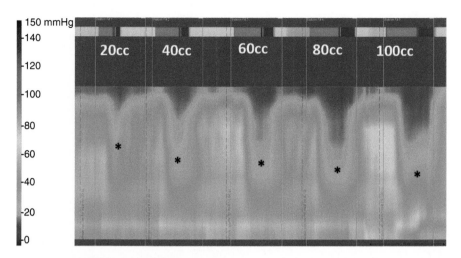

Figure 4.9 High-resolution anorectal manometry of a normal rectoanal inhibitory reflex (RAIR). The RAIR is a normal reflex mediated by the myenteric plexus. With sequentially larger volume of rectal balloon insufflation, the anal sphincter progressively relaxes (*asterisks*), as seen by the gradual change of the green color to blue on the color-pressure topography. This reflex generally starts on the rectal side of the anal canal and distributes caudally

and the pelvic floor muscles relax, and the subject generates higher pressure in the proximal rectum by recruiting abdominal wall muscle or performing a Valsalva maneuver to expel the stool. If it is not convenient, the EAS voluntarily contracts to further enhance stool continence.

This reflex can be evaluated during anorectal manometry by sequential inflation of the distal balloon mounted on the manometry catheter with progressively larger volumes. Three features can be observed. First, there should be a reduction in anal sphincter pressure with balloon inflation. The second feature is that the RAIR is graduated, so that anal relaxation is greater as balloon volume increases (Fig. 4.9). The third feature is that this graduated relaxation has a limit. When the volume is large, a reflex contraction occurs (Fig. 4.10). This is similar to the cough reflex and is meant to prevent overflow incontinence due to the arrival of a large volume of material in the lower rectum.

Classically, the RAIR is absent in individuals with aganglionosis (i.e., Hirschsprung's disease) and patients who have undergone low anterior resection or circular myotomy [14].

Simulated Defecation

During normal simulated defecation, the subject generates pressure in the proximal rectum, followed by appropriate relaxation of the pelvic floor muscles and anal sphincters. However, some patients may be afraid of incontinence or embarrassment

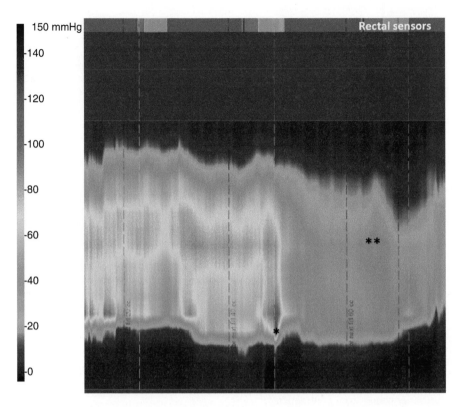

Figure 4.10   High-resolution anorectal manometry of voluntary external sphincter contraction in response to balloon inflation. With sequential balloon distention, the puborectalis and internal sphincter pressures decrease appropriately, seen as a change in color from red to green (*double asterisks*). This is a normal rectoanal inhibitory reflex (RAIR). The subject voluntarily contracts the external anal sphincter (*asterisk*) in response to the balloon inflation

during the anorectal manometry, which could lead to inappropriate contraction of the EAS or lack of appropriate relaxation (Fig. 4.11). This maneuver differs from usual defecation, as during anorectal manometry there is no rectal distension, owing to the absence of stool in the rectal vault. During normal defecation, the rectal pressure should exceed anal pressure to generate a pressure gradient for successful stool passage. Therefore, the normal rectoanal pressure gradient is positive and the rectoanal index is greater than 1, but a negative rectoanal pressure gradient is often seen in healthy individuals during simulated defecation. Hence, the utility of a negative rectoanal pressure gradient as a marker of defecatory disorder is unclear [15]. Sauter et al. [16] hypothesized that during simulated defecation, the catheter may come into contact with the wall of the anal canal, thereby producing "contact pressure" and spuriously raising the anal pressure. This effect can be partly explained by the subject's lateral position during anorectal manometry, which unnaturally eliminates the factor of gravity that supports defecation in the sitting position.

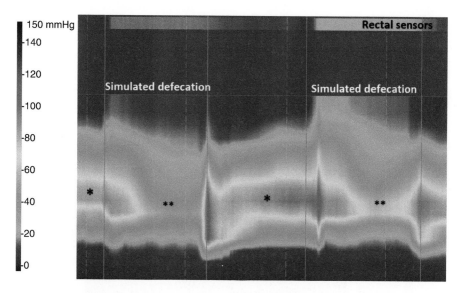

Figure 4.11 High-resolution anorectal manometry of normal simulated defecation. The rest-ing pressure of the anal sphincter (i.e., internal sphincter and puborectalis muscle) is approxi-mately 85 mm Hg, which is normal (*asterisk*). Upon simulated defecation, the puborectalis muscle and internal sphincter relax (*double asterisks*), as seen by a decrease in pressure to 40 mm Hg. During the first bear down, there is no rise in the intrarectal pressure (seen along the rectal sensors), as the subject does not elicit a Valsalva, suggesting a poor effort. Upon further guidance through the data acquisition, the subject recruits the abdominal muscles more effectively during the second simulated defecation, as shown by a rise in the pressure along the rectal sensors

Rectal Sensation

Rectal sensation is evaluated by sequentially inflating and deflating the balloon mounted on the manometry catheter. The balloon volumes at which the patient first reports sensation, urge to defecate, and maximum discomfort should be recorded. Typically, rectal hypersensitivity is seen in patients with urge incontinence, trau-matic or ulcerative proctitis, or hydrogen-predominant bacterial overgrowth, and sometimes in irritable bowel syndrome [17]. The presence of methane on a lactulose breath test appears to be associated with a relative rectal hyposensitivity during stepwise rectal distension [18]. In addition, rectal hyposensitivity can be seen in chronic idiopathic constipation, dyssynergic defecation, spinal injury, and neuropa-thy. On the other hand, the volume at the desire to defecate can be increased in patients with defecatory disorder and abnormal balloon expulsion [15]. In a study by Shin et al. [19], rectal hyposensitivity and inability to evacuate an intrarectal bal-loon are associated with poor response to biofeedback therapy for patients with dyssynergic defecation. Patients need some degree of rectal sensation in order to benefit from biofeedback therapy.

Bulbocavernosus Reflex (BCR)

Evaluation of the BCR can be an important add-on to anorectal manometry, especially in patients with known spinal cord injury. It is assessed by squeezing the glans penis or the clitoris, which causes an "anal wink" as the EAS briefly contracts. The intact reflex is easily appreciated on high-resolution anorectal manometry by transient contraction of the anal sphincters (Fig. 4.12).

The reflex is mediated through the pudendal nerve. In the case of a complete spinal lesion, the presence of BCR suggests an intact sacral (S2–S4) reflex arc; the loss of supraspinal inhibition suggests an upper motor neuron lesion. Th absence of BCR points to a lower motor neuron lesion [20].

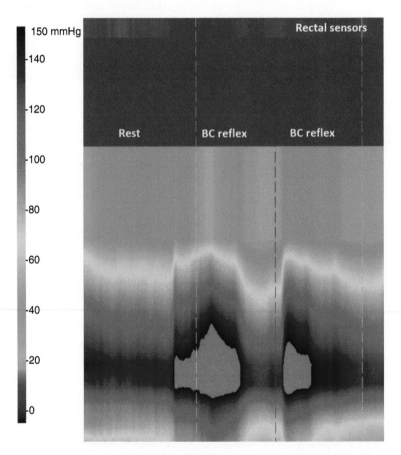

Figure 4.12 High-resolution anorectal manometry of the bulbocavernosus reflex. The bulbocavernosus (BC) reflex is an oligosynaptic sacral reflex that allows evaluation of the integrity of sacral sensory and motor fibers of the S2, S3, and S4 nerve roots and conus medullaris spinal nerves. The patient is asked to apply pressure to the glans penis or clitoris. The result is contraction of anal sphincters, seen as a rise in the pressure compared with the resting pressure. The reflex is intact in the study shown

Three-Dimensional Evaluation of Anal Sphincters

High-resolution anorectal manometry allows evaluation of the anorectal structure in both two and three dimensions (Fig. 4.13). Three-dimensional evaluation allows better assessment of the integrity of anal sphincters in cases of fecal incontinence and any abnormally high-pressure area that may be missed on a two-dimensional view (Figs. 4.14 and 4.15).

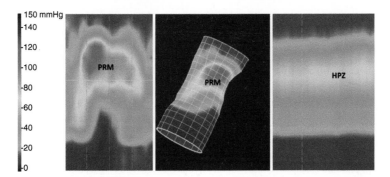

Figure 4.13 High-resolution three-dimensional anorectal manometry at rest. Anal sphincter pressure at rest in a normal, asymptomatic subject. **A,** A two-dimensional, cross-sectional view shows the horseshoe appearance of the puborectalis muscle (PRM). The PRM slings around the rectum at the anorectal junction posteriorly, and it is part of the pelvic floor girdle. At rest, the muscle is under tonic contraction, which is seen here as an area of high-pressure (*red color*). **B,** Three-dimensional view of the PRM and the internal anal sphincter. It is often difficult to separate these two structures from each other on anorectal manometry. **C,** High-resolution anorectal manometry of the resting anal sphincter pressure. The high-pressure zone (HPZ) corresponds to pressure generated by both the PRM and the internal anal sphincter at rest

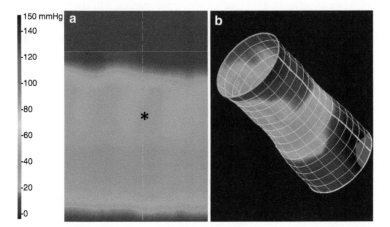

Figure 4.14 High-resolution anorectal manometry at rest. A, The resting anal sphincter pressure is somewhat diminished. In this two-dimensional view, there seems to be a defect in the internal anal sphincter resting pressure (*asterisk*). **B,** Switching to the three-dimensional view allows better assessment of the exact location of the sphincter defect, which seems to be a defect along the anterior aspect of the internal anal sphincter. The anorectal manometry finding of the anal sphincter defect should be corroborated by endoanal ultrasound

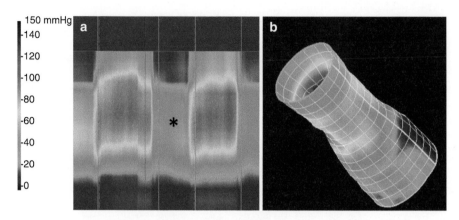

Figure 4.15 High-resolution anorectal manometry during simulated squeeze maneuver. A, A two-dimensional view of the simulated squeeze maneuver demonstrates normal contraction of the PRM and the external anal sphincter. Pressure is increased as compared with the baseline pressure (*asterisk*). **B,** A three-dimensional view of the simulated squeeze maneuver differentiates an asymmetrical area of high pressure generated by the contraction of the PRM, which acts as a sling around the posterior aspect of the distal rectum at the rectoanal junction. The rest of the circumferential high-pressure zone seems to be slightly hypotensive, suggesting a possible sphincter defect along the anterior/anterolateral aspect of the external anal sphincter. This finding should be confirmed by endoanal ultrasound

Abnormal High-Resolution Manometry

Ultraslow Wave

The ultraslow wave is a unique pattern that is occasionally seen in normal male patients [21] or in patients with anal pain or constipation. On anorectal manometry, these waves occur at a frequency of 1–1.5 cycles per minute and can be seen in a normal or hypertonic sphincter (Fig. 4.16). Their clinical significance is not exactly known. In a study by Eckardt et *al.* [22], patients with dyschezia had ultraslow waves, which were stimulated with anal squeeze and abolished with topical administration of isosorbide dinitrate.

Dyssynergic Defecation

The structure of the pelvic floor apparatus is complex. During normal defecation, the subject relaxes the pelvic floor muscles and anal sphincters while generating adequate proximal rectal pressure to expel the stool.

Patients with dyssynergic defecation often complain of incomplete evacuation, straining, passage of hard stool, and fewer than three stools per week [23]. When these symptoms are due to dyssynergic defecation, the patient cannot perform the coordinated movements that are required for normal stool passage. They may

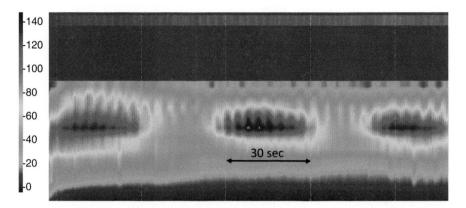

Figure 4.16 High-resolution anorectal manometry with ultraslow waves. This study was obtained at rest. The ultraslow waves are periodic oscillations in the anal canal, which occur over a period of 60 seconds. This pattern may be seen in subjects with a history of constipation or functional, painful anal canal pathology. These waves are considered to represent periodic hyperactivity of the internal anal sphincter, each lasting 30 seconds

experience impaired rectal contraction, paradoxical anal contraction, impaired anal relaxation, or a combination of mechanisms.

Rao et al. [23] demonstrated four patterns of dyssynergic defecation in constipated patients:

- Type I dyssynergia is seen when the patient generates an adequate propulsive force, seen as a rise in intrarectal pressure of at least 40 mm Hg, along with a paradoxical increase in anal sphincter pressure (Fig. 4.17).
- Type II is seen when the patient does not generate an adequate propulsive force, but there is again paradoxical anal contraction (Fig. 4.18).
- In type III, the subject can generate an adequate propulsive force, but there is either absent relaxation or incomplete (≤20%) anal sphincter relaxation (Fig. 4.19).
- Type IV is seen when the subject does not generate an adequate propulsive force, and relaxation of the anal sphincter is absent or incomplete (Fig. 4.20).

In addition, it is important to note that patients with dyssynergic defecation pattern may often have rectal hyposensation to balloon distension and the threshold for a desire to defecate [24]. One of the hypotheses explaining this finding is that rectal stool hoarding occurs, stretching the rectum. This stretched rectum needs greater balloon volumes to trigger the sensations associated with balloon distension. It is very important for those performing manometry to be aware of this phenomenon, as it can be mislabeled as potential neuropathy when it is not.

Dyssynergic defecation also commonly occurs in patients with ileal pouch anal anastomosis (IPAA) [6] and may present with various symptoms and signs such as diarrhea, fecal incontinence, constipation, rectal discomfort and non-healing pouch fistula (Fig. 4.21). Anal stricture should be ruled out prior to diagnosis of dyssynergic defcation in a patient with perianal Crohn's diesease or IPAA.

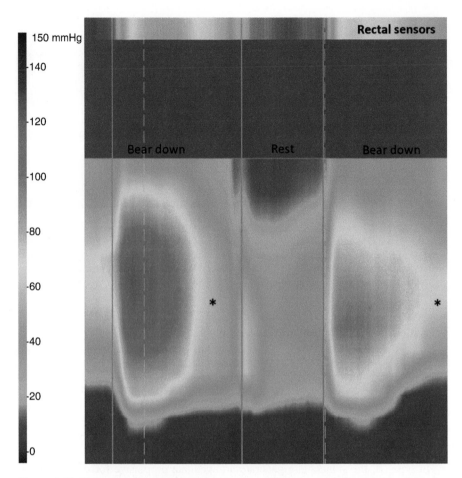

Figure 4.17 High-resolution anorectal manometry of dyssynergic defecation type I. During the simulated defecation, there is an appropriate rise in intrarectal (intra-abdominal) pressure, as the subject appropriately recruits the abdominal muscle, but there is a paradoxical contraction of anal canal musculature (PRM and external anal sphincter), as seen by the change in color from yellow (the basal pressure) to red (higher pressure). However, there is some relaxation at the end of each simulated defecation attempt (*asterisk*), close to the basal pressure. Therefore, this is an example of mild dyssynergic defecation type I

Hirschsprung's Disease

Hirschsprung's disease is a motor disorder of the gut, characterized by aganglionosis due to the failure of neural crest cells to migrate completely during fetal intestinal development. It can involve various length of the colon. Anorectal manometry may be required to diagnose ultrashort-segment Hirschsprung's disease, which can present as laxative-refractory constipation.

On anorectal manometry, patients with Hirschsprung's disease show an absence of rectoanal inhibitory reflex (RAIR) during balloon inflations, even with progressively larger volumes (Fig. 4.22).

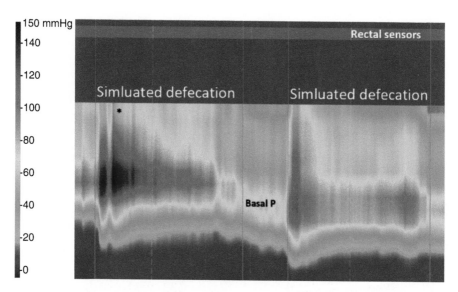

Figure 4.18 High-resolution anorectal manometry dyssynergic defecation type II. During the normal simulated defecation, there is a rise in intrarectal (intra-abdominal) pressure with Valsalva and a decrease in anal sphincter pressure. However, this anorectal manometry shows no rise in the intrarectal pressure sensors, and there is a paradoxical contraction of the PRM and external anal sphincter, compared with the resting pressure. There is also a rise in the pressure of the pelvic floor muscle (*asterisk*), although this is less contributory. This pattern is classified as type II dyssynergic defecation

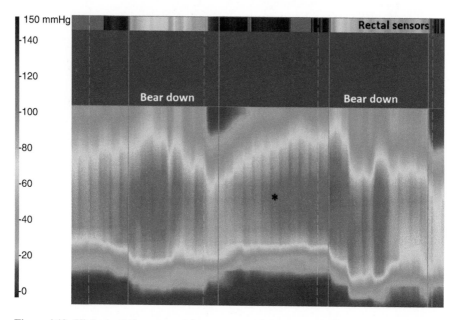

Figure 4.19 High-resolution anorectal manometry of dyssynergic defecation type III. There is an increase in intrarectal (i.e., intra-abdominal) pressure during simulated defecation, as noticeable by the rise in pressure in the rectal sensors during the simulated "bear down" maneuver. There is neither relaxation nor paradoxical contraction in the anal canal, compared with the baseline (*asterisk*). These are classic features of dyssynergic defecation type III

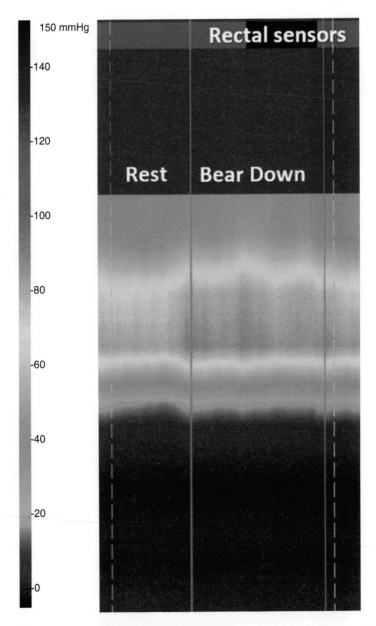

Figure 4.20 High-resolution anorectal manometry of dyssynergic defecation type IV. There is no increase in intrarectal (i.e., intra-abdominal) pressure along the rectal sensors. There is also a lack of anal sphincter relaxation on "bear down" when compared with the resting pressure. These findings are consistent with dyssynergic defecation type IV

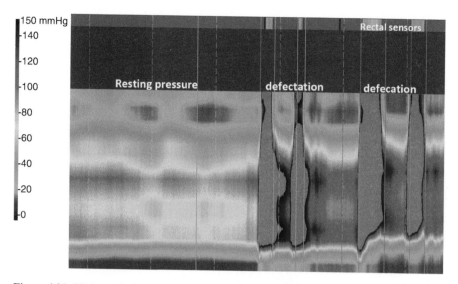

Figure 4.21 High resolution anorectal manometry of dyssynergic pouch. With all four simulated defecation maneuvers, the patient generates some intra-abdominal pressure, as seen along the rectal sensors. However, there is a paradoxical contraction of internal and external anal sphincters, as seen by a rise in pressure compared with the resting state. Therefore, this pattern is suggestive of defecatory dyssynergia

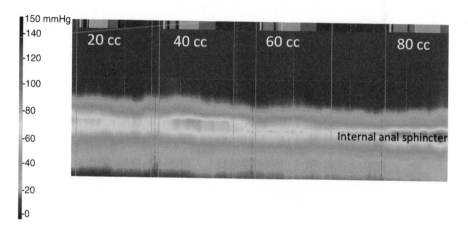

Figure 4.22 High-resolution anorectal manometry of absent rectoanal inhibitory reflex (RAIR) in Hirschsprung's disease. The balloon is inflated with sequentially larger volumes, but there is no relaxation of the internal anal sphincter, as demonstrated by the persistent band of pressure. Lack of relaxation of the internal anal sphincter with graded balloon distension is highly suggestive of Hirschsprung's disease because of the aganglionic segment of the colon. RAIR is a local reflex, mediated by the myenteric plexus. A similar pattern can be seen in patients with ileal-pouch anal anastomosis (IPAA), who lose RAIR in 50% of cases, as RAIR is driven mainly by the rectal interstitial cells of Cajal

Descending Perineum Syndrome

One of the under-recognized causes of constipation is descending perineum syndrome. The syndrome is recognized when the perineum balloons down during a "bear down" maneuver on the rectal exam [25]. These patients experience straining during defecation, incomplete evacuation, mucus discharge, anal outlet bleeding secondary to a solitary rectal ulcer associated with anterior rectal wall prolapse, and even hemorrhoids or anal fissures. Patients may also experience poorly localized deep perineal pain, urine and/or stool urge incontinence, or vaginal prolapse. Excessive perineal descent can lead to the development of fecal incontinence over time by inducing nerve injuries to the pudendal nerve and sacral roots, as it reduces the rectoanal angle, which in turn stretches these nerves [26]. The pudendal nerve innervates the external sphincter, and the sacral roots tonically innervate the puborectalis muscle [27]. Normal perineal descent is 1–3.5 cm, with 3.9 cm being the upper limit of normal. Therefore, any perineal descent greater than 4 cm is considered exaggerated and abnormal [28]. Figure 4.23 shows anorectal manometry of a patient with excessive perineal descent.

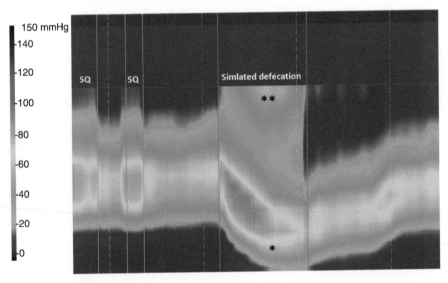

Figure 4.23 High-resolution anorectal manometry of a patient with descending perineum syndrome. This patient has normal squeeze pressure (SQ), as demonstrated by increased pressure compared with the baseline, the resting anal sphincter pressure. During the simulated defecation, there is a significant descent of the perineum along the manometry catheter. These findings can be corroborated with a defecography study. Descending perineum syndrome can be seen in the setting of multiple pregnancies or joint hypermobility syndromes, especially Ehlers-Danlos type III. Pressure from the rectal mucosa coming into contact with the probe (*double asterisks*) is a result of the significant descent of the pelvic space. Upon relaxation, the anal sphincter slowly returns to the baseline position

Anal Sphincter Defects

Anal sphincter defects are one of the most common reasons for anorectal manometry. Their many causes include iatrogenic causes such as previous sphincterectomy and hemorrhoidectomy, but the most common are pelvic trauma or obstetrical injuries (episiotomy, poor alignment of suture during repair of episiotomy, perineal tears). Interestingly, because there are redundant continence mechanisms such as the puborectalis muscle, obstetrical injuries may not manifest as incontinence for decades, revealing themselves with age and puborectalis dysfunction or fatigue. Urgency and incontinence of stool then become alarming symptoms that patients describe (Fig. 4.24).

Anorectal manometry is very helpful to identify weakness in the sphincter. Three-dimensional high-definition manometry can help to identify the location and size of the sphincter injury. In many instances, puborectalis weakness can also be seen. Most cases of anorectal injury or weakness are found anteriorly or anterolaterally [29]. When large defects are discovered, it is best to complement these manometry findings with endoanal ultrasound or pelvic MRI prior to any consideration of surgical repair.

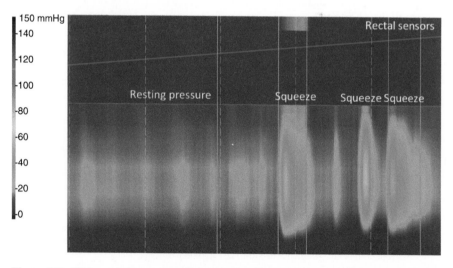

Figure 4.24 High-resolution anorectal manometry of a patient with fecal incontinence after pelvic radiation. The resting pressure of the internal anal sphincter is significantly diminished. The patient can generate higher pressures (predominantly generated by the external anal sphincter) during "squeezing simulation," but overall, the squeezing pressure is low

References

1. Lee YY, Erdogan A, Yu S, Dewitt A, Rao SSC. Anorectal manometry in defecatory disorders: a comparative analysis of high-resolution pressure topography and waveform manometry. J Neurogastroenterol Motil. 2018;24:460–8.
2. Rao SSC. Rectal exam: yes, it can and should be done in a busy practice! Am J Gastroenterol. 2018;113:635–8.
3. Rao SS, Azpiroz F, Diamant N, Enck P, Tougas G, Wald A. Minimum standards of anorectal manometry. Neurogastroenterol Motil. 2002;14:553–9.
4. Shah ED, Farida JD, Menees S, Baker JR, Chey WD. Examining balloon expulsion testing as an office-based, screening test for dyssynergic defecation: a systematic review and meta-analysis. Am J Gastroenterol. 2018;113:1613–20.
5. Rao SS, Hasler WL. Can high-resolution anorectal manometry shed new light on defecatory disorders? Gastroenterology. 2013;144:263–5.
6. Rezaie A, Gu P, Kaplan GG, Pimentel M, Al-Darmaki AK. Dyssynergic defecation in inflammatory bowel disease: a systematic review and meta-analysis. Inflamm Bowel Dis. 2018;24:1065–73.
7. Bharucha AE. Pelvic floor: anatomy and function. Neurogastroenterol Motil. 2006;18:507–19.
8. Carrington EV, Brokjaer A, Craven H, Zarate N, Horrocks EJ, Palit S, et al. Traditional measures of normal anal sphincter function using high-resolution anorectal manometry (HRAM) in 115 healthy volunteers. Neurogastroenterol Motil. 2014;26:625–35.
9. Opazo A, Aguirre E, Saldana E, Fantova MJ, Clave P. Patterns of impaired internal anal sphincter activity in patients with anal fissure. Colorectal Dis. 2013;15:492–9.
10. Lee HJ, Jung KW, Han S, Kim JW, Park SK, Yoon IJ, et al. Normal values for high-resolution anorectal manometry/topography in a healthy Korean population and the effects of gender and body mass index. Neurogastroenterol Motil. 2014;26:529–37.
11. Azpiroz F, Enck P, Whitehead WE. Anorectal functional testing: review of collective experience. Am J Gastroenterol. 2002;97:232–40.
12. Fox M, Schwizer W, Menne D, Stutz B, Fried M, Thumshirn M. The physical properties of rectal contents have effects on anorectal continence: insights from a study into the cause of fecal spotting on orlistat. Dis Colon Rectum. 2004;47:2147–56.
13. Miller R, Bartolo DC, Cervero F, Mortensen NJ. Anorectal sampling: a comparison of normal and incontinent patients. Br J Surg. 1988;75:44–7.
14. Sangwan YP, Solla JA. Internal anal sphincter: advances and insights. Dis Colon Rectum. 1998;41:1297–311.
15. Ratuapli SK, Bharucha AE, Noelting J, Harvey DM, Zinsmeister AR. Phenotypic identification and classification of functional defecatory disorders using high-resolution anorectal manometry. Gastroenterology. 2013;144:314–22 e2.
16. Sauter M, Heinrich H, Fox M, Misselwitz B, Halama M, Schwizer W, et al. Toward more accurate measurements of anorectal motor and sensory function in routine clinical practice: validation of high-resolution anorectal manometry and Rapid Barostat Bag measurements of rectal function. Neurogastroenterol Motil. 2014;26:685–95.
17. Mulak A, Paradowski L. Anorectal function and dyssynergic defecation in different subgroups of patients with irritable bowel syndrome. Int J Colorectal Dis. 2010;25:1011–6.
18. Rezaie A. Methane on breath test predicts altered rectal sensation during high resolution anorectal manometry. Gastroenterology. 2014;146:S-721.
19. Shin JK, Cheon JH, Kim ES, Yoon JY, Lee JH, Jeon SM, et al. Predictive capability of anorectal physiologic tests for unfavorable outcomes following biofeedback therapy in dyssynergic defecation. J Korean Med Sci. 2010;25:1060–5.
20. Previnaire JG. The importance of the bulbocavernosus reflex. Spinal Cord Ser Cases. 2018;4:2.
21. Rao SS, Read NW, Stobart JA, Haynes WG, Benjamin S, Holdsworth CD. Anorectal contractility under basal conditions and during rectal infusion of saline in ulcerative colitis. Gut. 1988;29:769–77.

22. Eckardt VF, Schmitt T, Bernhard G. Anal ultra slow waves: a smooth muscle phenomenon associated with dyschezia. Dig Dis Sci. 1997;42:2439–45.

23. Rao SS, Tuteja AK, Vellema T, Kempf J, Stessman M. Dyssynergic defecation: demographics, symptoms, stool patterns, and quality of life. J Clin Gastroenterol. 2004;38:680–5.

24. Rao SS, Welcher KD, Leistikow JS. Obstructive defecation: a failure of rectoanal coordination. Am J Gastroenterol. 1998;93:1042–50.

25. Henry MM, Parks AG, Swash M. The pelvic floor musculature in the descending perineum syndrome. Br J Surg. 1982;69:470–2.

26. Parks AG, Porter NH, Hardcastle J. The syndrome of the descending perineum. Proc R Soc Med. 1966;59:477–82.

27. Harewood GC, Coulie B, Camilleri M, Rath-Harvey D, Pemberton JH. Descending perineum syndrome: audit of clinical and laboratory features and outcome of pelvic floor retraining. Am J Gastroenterol. 1999;94:126–30.

28. Pezim ME, Pemberton JH, Levin KE, Litchy WJ, Phillips SF. Parameters of anorectal and colonic motility in health and in severe constipation. Dis Colon Rectum. 1993;36:484–91.

29. Rezaie A, Iriana S, Pimentel M, Murrell Z, Fleshner P, Zaghiyan K. Can three-dimensional high-resolution anorectal manometry detect anal sphincter defects in patients with faecal incontinence? Colorectal Dis. 2017;19(5):468–75.

Chapter 5
Basic Principles of Ambulatory pH Monitoring and Impedance

Introduction

Gastroesophageal reflux disease (GERD) has a worldwide prevalence of 8–33%, involving both sexes and all age groups [1]. Based on the Montreal consensus definition, GERD is the reflux of stomach contents causing troublesome symptoms and/or complications [2]. High scores on the available questionnaires, such as GerdQ, have shown to be predictive of abnormal pH monitoring off proton pump inhibitor (PPI) therapy, but overall they have modest accuracy in diagnosing GERD [3]. The sensitivity of GERD questionnaires in diagnosing GERD has been found to be 62%, similar to the sensitivity of 63% for family physicians and 67% for gastroenterologists; the specificities were 67%, 63%, and 70%, respectively. However, the questionnaire was not associated with an abnormal pH test in any patients using PPI therapy [4]. Therefore, reflux testing is necessary in the evaluation of patients with typical and atypical symptoms of GERD. It should be emphasized that while the current ambulatory systems are the best available test for pH monitoring, they are by no means considered as the gold standard. Various systems have many limitations and advantages and disadvantages, which are briefly discussed throughout this chapter. Overall, the sensitivity of pH monitoring in erosive esophagitis approximates 77–100%, and the specificity is 85–100%. The sensitivity of the catheter improves to 91% with the addition of impedance, but it is notable that in those with normal upper endoscopy, the sensitivity is less than 70% [5].

According to the Lyon Consensus [6], pathological reflux in patients with bothersome symptoms, especially in those with typical symptoms of heartburn and regurgitation, is defined as conclusive evidence of reflux esophagitis (Los Angeles classification C or D), a long segment of Barrett's esophagus or peptic stricture on endoscopy, or distal esophageal acid exposure time greater than 6% on the ambulatory pH or pH-impedance monitoring. A normal endoscopy does not rule out reflux, highlighting the necessity to arrange pH monitoring with or without impedance to complete the workup in patients with symptoms typical of reflux.

© Springer Nature Switzerland AG 2020
S. Moosavi et al., *Atlas of High-Resolution Manometry, Impedance, and pH Monitoring*, https://doi.org/10.1007/978-3-030-27241-8_5

Table 5.1 Indications for pH Monitoring

Preoperative work-up for antireflux surgery
Work-up in patients with typical or atypical GERD symptoms with normal upper endoscopy
PPI-refractory GERD
Recurrent belching, cough, and work-up of rumination syndrome (with the latter, in conjunction with prolonged esophageal manometry)
Emerging role in preoperative work-up of lung transplantation

GERD—gastroesophageal reflux disease; PPI—proton pump inhibitor

A normal-appearing esophagus on the upper endoscopy, in conjunction with distal acid exposure time less than 4% and fewer than 40 reflux episodes on pH-impedance monitoring when the patient is off PPI therapy makes GERD very unlikely. In patients who have normal upper endoscopy but typical symptoms of reflux, pH monitoring remains the most informative diagnostic test for GERD evaluation (though not perfect), especially if these patients that are being considered for antireflux surgery. Contemporary data suggest that antireflux procedures for GERD are as effective as medical therapy and should be offered to appropriately selected patients by experienced, skilled surgeons. Therefore, pH monitoring and esophageal manometry have become an integral part of the preoperative workup for this patient population [7], as noted in Table 5.1. In addition, current guidelines also recommend pH monitoring in the evaluation of patients with GERD that is refractory to PPI therapy (defined as a trial of double the standard dose of PPI for 8 weeks), as well as in those with a questionable diagnosis of GERD [8].

Technique

The field of GERD has been revolutionized over the past several decades. In 1958, Tuttle and Grossman introduced a technique that was able to recognize the pH gradient between the esophagus and stomach. In 1974, Johnson and Demeester established a landmark study with a technique to measure esophageal pH after studying normal subjects and patients with reflux symptoms, which allowed them to introduce normal values for 24-hour pH monitoring [9].

The pH catheters have also evolved with the advancement in this field. Currently, a variety of different catheters are available. Single-sensor catheter-based pH probes allow for traditional acid reflux measurements in the distal esophagus. In addition, the newer catheter-based ambulatory pH monitoring allows the addition of impedance to pH monitoring in multichannel intraluminal impedance pH monitoring (MII-pH). Impedance detects variable resistance to current flow with a bolus of air, liquid, or food through a series of paired electrodes. These electrodes can detect substance distribution, composition, and clearance times. The impedance sensors are located at 3, 5, 7, 9, 15, and 17 cm above the lower esophageal sphincter (LES), measured manometrically [10]. Therefore, the MII-pH catheter allows the assessment of both acidic and non-acidic reflux (i.e., weakly acidic and alkaline reflux), as well as liquid, air, or mixed refluxates. This system may be valuable in the work-up of patients with PPI-refractory or atypical GERD symptoms [11]. These latter patients, experience symptoms related to non-acidic liquid bolus reflux, events that can precipitate heartburn but are more often attributed to extra-esophageal manifestations such as aspiration.

Dual-channel 24-hour pH monitoring catheters have advantages over single-sensor devices. They allow data collection from both the proximal and distal esophagus. If abnormal acid exposure is detected at both the upper and lower pH probes, it is inferred that it can produce or be associated with laryngopharyngeal symptoms, but if acid is measured only in the upper probe, the relationship of reflux to laryngopharyngeal symptoms is less certain [12]. Therefore, this method may be informative in patients with refractory cough, throat clearing, globus sensation, or sore throat. One pitfall with these devices is that the fixed distances between the pH sensors result in misplacement of the proximal probe in roughly 45% of patients [13]. In addition, dual pH/impedance catheters with variable distances between the pH sensors (12, 15, 19, or 22 cm) are available. Following esophageal manometry and accurate assessment of the distance from the nares to the LES and upper esophageal sphincter (UES), the use of dual pH/impedance catheters can decrease the rate of misplacement of the proximal pH sensors. This is especially useful in placement of catheters used to detect laryngopharyngeal reflux (LPR).

Symptoms of LPR are often treated empirically with acid suppression, but establishing the symptomatic pharyngeal reflux in patients with LPR is less straightforward. With previously available catheters, non-acid reflux and pepsin may have not been measured, but we now know that non-acid reflux and pepsin play a significant role in the pathophysiology of LPR. PH/impedance catheters that extend only 15 cm above the LES will not capture all potentially deleterious events [14]. There is evidence that antireflux surgery is successful for LPR in patients selected using a hypopharyngeal-esophageal multichannel impedance catheter with dual pH to detect true LPR in patients with chronic cough [15].

Multichannel intraluminal impedance and pH testing (MII-pH) is considered the current gold standard in reflux testing, with validated criteria such as more than 31 impedance events in the proximal esophagus (15 cm above the LES or acid events beyond the UES) as diagnostic criteria for LPR [16]. Normative data suggest that as few as two pharyngeal impedance events in 24 hours may be abnormal [17]. The hypopharyngeal-esophageal multichannel impedance/pH (HEMII-pH) testing catheters are equipped with two pH sensors (one used to detect LPR at the UES and the other to detect GERD proximal to the LES) and eight esophageal impedance electrodes located above the UES and within the esophageal body. Three sizes of catheters with the pre-determined distances of 15 cm, 19 cm, and 22 cm between the pH probes are available. The impedance electrodes flank both the proximal and distal pH probe. For example, in catheters that have pH probes 15 cm apart, impedance electrodes are 1 and 3 cm below and 1, 3, and 5 cm above the distal pH probe. In these catheters, other impedance electrodes are located 1 and 3 cm below and 1 cm above the proximal pH probe. In catheters with pH probes 19 or 22 cm apart, impedance electrodes are 1 cm above and 1 and 3 cm below the distal pH proble. In these catheters, other impedances electrodes are 1 cm above and 2, 5, and 7 cm below the proximal pH probe. The proximal pH probe is placed within 1 cm of the UES as measured by esophageal manometry. Given these set catheter lengths, the distal pH probe may not necessarily be placed 5 cm proximal to the LES.

"Pharyngeal" reflux is defined by events recorded by the hypopharyngeal imped- ance sensor electrode pairs, positioned within and just above the UES. Two or more events at the hypopharyngeal pair are considered abnormal. In a study by Borges et al. [18], 81% of patients with LPR symptoms tested positive for abnormal pha- ryngeal reflux based on the previously published cut-off of two or more pharyngeal impedance events being outside normative values in 24 hours; 92% had six or more events in 24 hours detected by impedance sensors just below the UES, in those who failed to improve with PPI therapy. In addition, it was shown that traditional imped- ance criteria for both distal and proximal esophageal reflux up to 14 cm above the LES were not reliable in excluding abnormal pharyngeal reflux. Therefore, this study supports the use of HEMII-pH (with pharyngeal impedance sensors) in the evaluation of patients with refractory symptoms and highlights our current lack of understanding about what constitutes a true positive HEMII-pH test. When a belch or swallow accompanies a reflux event, however, the pharyngeal events become less clear or reliable, so the proximal esophageal event just below the UES may prove to be more reliable than actual pharyngeal events. More work is required to evaluate this suspicion [18].

In the 1990s, a wireless implantable capsule (Bravo™ probe, Given imaging, Shoreview, MN, USA) system was first introduced. The most recent generation of these wireless capsules is capable of recording data longer than 24 hours, up to 96 hours. In a study by Prakash and Clouse [19], extending pH recording time to 2 days with the wireless pH monitoring system increased the likelihood of detecting reflux disease in patients, particularly those with atypical symptoms and day-to-day varia- tion of reflux. This wireless system is more easily tolerated by patients. Rarely, patients may complain of chest pain or dysphagia, which may require repeat endos- copy for the capsule removal. The disadvantage of this system is that it can only record the distal esophageal pH and may dislodge prematurely. This can be seen by rapid drop of pH to less than 2, compatible with the capsule dropping in the stom- ach, followed by rapid pH rise to >8, which happens when the pH capsule transi- tions into the small bowel. It is important to recognize premature capsule dislodgement to avoid misinterpreting the collected data.

The Bravo™ wireless pH monitoring capsule is contraindicated in those with bleeding diathesis or anticoagulation, esophageal varices, severe reflux esophagitis, stricture, history of bowel obstruction, a pacemaker, or a defibrillator. The trocar needle in the Bravo capsule is made of stainless steel, so caution is required for patients with known allergies to chromium, nickel, copper, cobalt, and iron. On the other hand, the new longer measurement gives the clinician the ability to record pH monitoring both off and on PPI therapy during the same capsule insertion, which cannot be done with 24 hour pH or pH/impedance catheters.

Another catheter available for assessment of extra-esophageal GERD symptoms is the Restech pH-catheter device (Respiratory Technology Corp., San Diego, CA).

This is a pharyngeal pH probe designed to detect aerosolized and liquid acid reflux. However, studies have shown that pharyngeal reflux occurring without events detected by esophageal pH-impedance probes used simultaneously is more suggestive of a non-reflux cause of pH drop. Considering these limitations, a recent consensus from an international group of experts considered that there is no clear evidence that dual pH probe alone or measurement of airway and pharyngeal pH can be recommended to diagnose gastroesophageal reflux episodes extending to the pharynx [20, 21].

Performance of Ambulatory pH Monitoring

Patients are asked to fast for 4–6 hours before pH monitoring testing, to reduce the risk of vomiting during the catheter insertion. In the case of wireless capsule pH monitoring, patients usually require upper endoscopy for the capsule placement. In some centers, Bravo™ capsule placement has been done transnasally without endoscopy, but the delivery system of this device is rather bulky, and patients may not tolerate its passage through the nares. The pH catheter or capsule is calibrated to pH of 4 and 7 ex vivo prior to the insertion, following the manufacturer's instructions.

For the ambulatory pH/impedance catheter, the tip is placed 5 cm above the gastroesophageal junction, measured manometrically, because up to 2 cm of movement in either direction can be expected with swallowing and head movement, and this location reduces catheter migration into the stomach [27]. For the Bravo™, the capsule is attached to the esophageal mucosa 6 cm above the squamocolumnar junction identified during endoscopy (or 9 cm above the upper border of the manometrically defined LES from the nostrils), or 6 cm proximal to rugal folds in cases of patients with Barrett's esophagus; this corresponds with 5 cm above the LES on the pH catheter [28, 29]. For catheter-based pH monitoring, the external lead is attached to a recording device, whereas the Bravo™ capsule is a wireless system that transmits radiofrequency data to an external recorder. In both instances, collected data are downloaded at the conclusion of the study to the vendor-provided computer software for further analysis.

During the pH testing, patients are instructed to keep a food diary, record their symptoms, and document their upright and recumbent positions. Patients are asked to continue their regular daily activities, to ensure that the pH monitoring is truly representative of their typical daily routine. Subjects should avoid drinking fluid with pH <5 or pH >6 or snacking frequently between meals, although there is no consensus in the literature regarding the exact dietary restrictions during the pH monitoring; dietary instructions likely vary among different centers. Patients should avoid submerging the recorder in water and should keep the recorder close (within 5 feet) to avoid gaps in the recorded measurements due to poor communication [11].

For adequate impressions, the study should be recorded for at least 16 hours. Mealtimes are excluded, as during data analysis, most software excludes the period 2 hours after each meal. The software generates the preliminary data for further interpretation. Overall, the automated analysis of pH impedance studies is adequate for acid reflux events, but often overestimates nonacidic or weakly acidic events. Therefore, manual review of the </=2 minutes preceding each symptom event in pH impedance studies is usually necessary.

Establishing a relationship between chronic cough and reflux is challenging, even though chronic cough may be associated with weakly acidic reflux. The use of impedance-pH rather than pH alone is favored, and the use of a cough detector may improve accuracy [22–26]. (Of note, when cough detectors are used, studies have shown a lower rate of accurate patient reporting [21]). With the added ability to measure nonacid reflux events, including the consistency of refluxate and its height as well as bolus transit, multichannel impedance/pH (MII-pH) catheters have been preferentially used to evaluate patients with atypical GERD symptoms, including asthma and reflux laryngitis. In addition, these catheters may be helpful in assessing patients with belching and those suspected of having rumination syndrome. Because rumination and GERD may look similar on pH monitoring, these patients need complementary evaluation, usually with prolonged esophageal manometry of about 30–90 minutes with a provoking or standardized meal. It is important to note that the wireless system (Bravo™ Capsule) cannot assess non-acidic reflux given its lack of impedance information.

The most updated consensus on ambulatory reflux monitoring for diagnosis of GERD was published by Roman et al. [20] regarding patients who have persistent symptoms suggestive of GERD, mainly heartburn and regurgitation, history of moderate to severe reflux esophagitis (LA classification C or D), Barrett's mucosa, peptic stricture, or prior history of positive pH testing. The recommendation is to perform 24-hour impedance monitoring on double-dose PPI to ensure adequate GERD control. On the other hand, in patients who have normal upper endoscopy without esophagitis (grade C or D), Barrett's mucosa, or peptic stricture; those who have atypical or PPI-refractory symptoms; or those planning antireflux surgery, pH monitoring should be performed with no PPI therapy for 7 days before the test.

Even though various catheters have been developed, the principles of pH monitoring and test interpretation remain relatively unchanged. In the study by DeMeester and Johnson [1, 30], a composite scoring system, the DeMeester score, was introduced to quantify acid exposure using six pH parameters, including total time of pH <4, upright time of pH <4, supine time of pH <4, number of reflux episodes, number of reflux episodes lasting for 5 minutes or longer, and the length of the longest episode in minutes. In addition to these six parameters, the calculated DeMeester score, total test duration, as well as duration in upright and supine positions and in postprandial periods are reported. If the DeMeester score is less than 14.72, then the likelihood of pathologic acid exposure is considered low, using this method. If the score is positive (i.e., ≥14.72), then the study is suggestive of positive acid exposure. It is also important then to assess the study for reflux pattern, during both the supine and upright position. Prandial reflux episodes are eliminated, so it is critical for patients to mark both start and finish times of meals in the diary. Table 5.2 outlines the normative values for different parameters evaluated through 24-hour pH monitoring. The proximal values are reported at 15 centimeters proximal to the LES [24].

Another important parameter is acid exposure time (AET), which is calculated through a cumulative summation of time when esophageal pH is below 4 over the

Table 5.2 Normative Values for Parameters Evaluated Through 24-Hour pH Monitoring

Value	Normal
Time spent in reflux	
% Time in reflux—total	<6%
% Time in reflux—upright	<9.7%
% Time in reflux—supine	<2.1%
% Time in reflux-postprandial	N/A
DeMeester score	<14.72
Acid reflux episodes	≤55
Weakly acidic reflux episodes	≤26
Non-acid reflux episodes	≤1
Total reflux episodes	≤72
Proximal acid reflux	<28 (total) <25 (upright) <2 (recumbent)
Proximal weakly acidic reflux	<12 (total) <11 (upright) <1 (recumbent)
Proximal nonacid reflux	<1 (total) <1 (upright) 0 (recumbent)
Proximal total reflux	<31 (total) <29 (upright) <3 (recumbent)

study duration. A general inspection of the pH study should be performed to exclude any artifacts that may be due to catheter displacement or wireless capsule dislodgement, which could spuriously increase the AET by sensors in the acidic stomach [31]. By consensus, the AET is the favored metric used to designate esophageal acid burden. In general, an elevated AET predicts a positive response to a PPI trial [26, 32, 33] and symptom outcome following antireflux therapy [34, 35]. According to the consensus, patients who have grade C or D esophagitis and/or peptic stricture and/or Barrett's esophagus on upper endoscopy, or AET greater than 6%, or more than 80 reflux events in 24 hours, have pathologic GERD. On the other hand, those who have normal upper endoscopy and AET less than 4% are very unlikely to have pathologic GERD. Those who have normal endoscopy or mild reflux esophagitis (grade A or B) or AET of 4–6% fall in a "grey zone," and further evidence may be required to evaluate pathologic GERD, including the number of reflux events, baseline impedance, or biopsy for microscopic esophagitis [20].

The pH-Impedance performed with the patient "on" PPI therapy allows further evaluation of non-acid reflux, subclassified as weakly acidic (pH >4 and <7) or weakly alkaline (pH >7), which is found to be particularly important in PPI non-responders. It is also a valuable test to assess in those with significant Barrett's esophagus or severe erosive esophagitis, to assess whether there is adequate acid control. Performing pH monitoring "off" PPI therapy should be considered in patients with low pre-test probability of having GERD, patients with pending anti-reflux surgery but no prior objective documentation of pathologic reflux, or patients with PPI-refractory symptoms without prior objective evaluation for GERD. Given that pH monitoring is far from a perfect test, it is pertinent to consider the patient's history of presenting illness when interpreting the pH monitoring and implementing a management plan [5].

Patients are asked to keep a diary of symptoms, which allows the interpreter to assess symptom correlation measures such as the symptom index (SI), symptom sensitivity index (SSI), and symptom association probability (SAP) [11]. Both pH and combined MII-pH monitoring provide information to assess the temporal association between symptoms and reflux episodes. The automated recorder allows the patient to push the relevant buttons as set up for specific symptoms before the pH monitoring begins. The recorder is set to the most bothersome or dominant symptoms. Keeping the diary will allow the technician to further cross-reference the accuracy of recorded symptoms with the written diary and fill in any gaps that patients may have forgotten to enter in the recorder. The time window to be used for symptoms following a reflux event is 2 minutes.

Various parameters have been used to evaluate symptom correlation. The SI and SAP have been proposed as clinically useful tools to assess whether a particular symptom is associated with a reflux event. The SSI, defined as the ratio of symptomatic reflux episodes divided by the total number of reflux episodes, has fallen out of favor, as it does not take into account the total number of symptomatic episodes. Therefore, it is not discussed in this chapter.

SI is the number of symptoms associated with a reflux event divided by the total number of symptoms. SI greater than 50% is considered positive, with a sensitivity of 93% and specificity of 71% for GERD [36]. However, this parameter does not take into consideration the total number of reflux episodes. Therefore, if one symptom occurs during a reflux event "by chance", the SI could be 100%. The outcome of symptom association analysis is more reliable when the symptoms occur in at least three events during the test [20].

SAP is a complex calculation of all symptoms and reflux episodes, by creating a 2×2 contingency table and using the Fisher's exact test P value. An SAP that is greater than 95% is considered positive; it indicates that the observed association between symptoms and reflux events occurs by chance less than 5% of the time, so it is a measure of probability [36]. It is generally thought that the SAP is the most statistically valid parameter [5], but the sensitivity of SAP in assessing GERD is 65.2%, and its specificity is 73.3% [37].

As these two metrics assess distinct aspects of pH monitoring, they cannot be compared with each other; in fact, they complement each other, and the combination of both positive SI and SAP provides the best evidence of clinically relevant symptoms–reflux association. Studies have shown that SI and SAP can be discordant, however, especially when the frequency of symptoms is very high or very low [38]. Both the SI and SAP have complementary value in data analysis and cannot be directly compared to each other. The consensus recommends evaluating SI only if SAP is positive [20].

Various aspects of pH monitoring and impedance are reviewed in Figures 5.1 through 5.16, including the use of pH/impedance catheters or a dual pH catheter to determine the nature of reflux (Figs. 5.1–5.7), detection of LPR (Fig. 5.8) or suspicion of a hiatal hernia (Fig. 5.9), assessment of PPI response (Figs. 5.10 and 5.11), evaluation of aerophagia and belching (Figs. 5.12–5.14), and malfunctions of monitoring systems (Figs. 5.15 and 5.16).

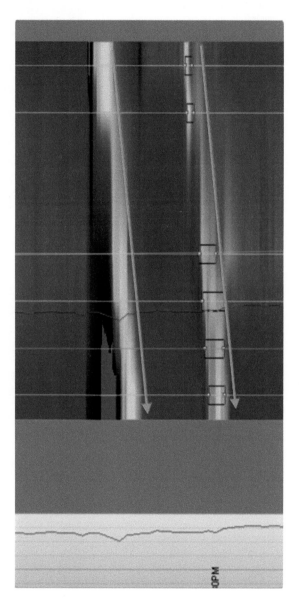

Figure 5.1 pH-monitoring tracing of two normal swallows with a pH/impedance catheter. There is an antegrade propagation of normal swallows, as evident by aboral drop in impedance. Considering that the liquid bolus contains electrolytes, the impedance drops (lower impedance appears white). Impedance is inversely proportional to resistance to conductivity between the two adjacent impedance sensors. Therefore, the liquid bolus causes a decrease in impedance, while gas interferes with conductivity between the adjacent impedance sensors and causes an increase in impedance (higher impedance appears black or grey). The *orange arrows* show the slope of the swallow. Note the lack of a significant drop in the pH measurement (*red line*), meaning that non-acidic material was consumed

Figure 5.2 pH-monitoring tracing of an episode of acid reflux with a pH/impedance catheter. There is a "triangular" drop in impedance. The gastric refluxate moves retrograde into the distal esophagus, followed by subsequent antegrade clearance from the esophagus. The distal pH sensor registered a pH less than 4. Therefore, this is a liquid acidic refluxate.

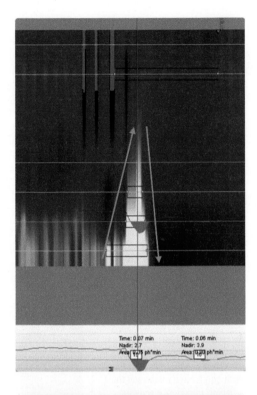

Figure 5.3 pH-monitoring tracing of a more prolonged episode of non-acid reflux with a pH/impedance catheter. There is a "triangular" drop in impedance. The gastric refluxate moves retrograde into the distal esophagus, and subsequently clears the esophagus. The distal pH sensor registered a pH greater than 4, so this is a liquid, non-acidic refluxate (weakly acidic reflux)

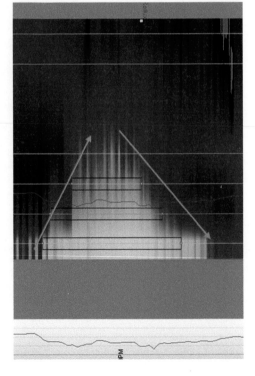

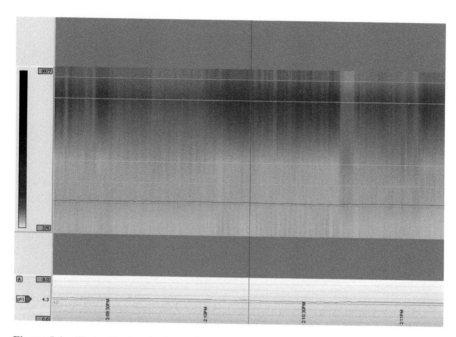

Figure 5.4 pH-monitoring tracing using pH/impedance catheter. There is a baseline low impedance, as depicted by pale blue/white color. This pattern is generally seen in patients with impaired esophageal mucosal integrity, such as reflux esophagitis, Barrett's esophagus, eosinophilic esophagitis, or an underlying esophageal motility disorder, especially when the baseline impedance is less than 500 ohm. It can also be seen in esophageal dysmotility, including achalasia, severe ineffective esophageal dysmotility, and aperistaltic esophagus. Given the low baseline impedance, which may be due to fluid retention in the esophagus, the sensitivity of the test for detecting non-acidic reflux on impedance could be affected and the study may underestimate the non-acid or weakly alkaline reflux episodes.

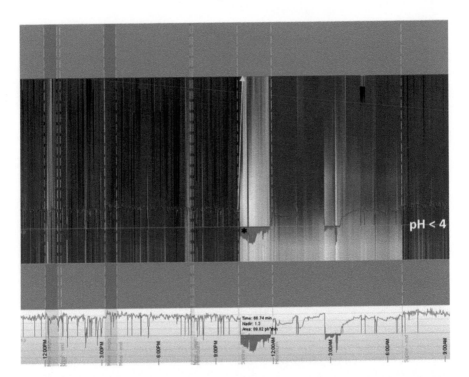

Figure 5.5   24-hour pH/impedance monitoring of a patient with persistent heartburn despite daily dosing of 40 mg of omeprazole. As seen in the distal pH sensor, there is a drop in pH below 4 with the onset of supine position (*asterisk*), as well as retrograde movement of gastric content (*yellow arrow*), associated with a drop in impedance (*white color*) extending to the proximal esophagus. Therefore, the retrograde refluxate is composed of pure liquid. This reflux episode lasts longer than an hour, and eventually the impedance recovers to baseline, as the refluxate is cleared from the esophagus. There are two shorter episodes of acid reflux around 3:00 AM. The patient did not record symptoms associated with any of these episodes. These findings are compatible with night-time acid reflux breakthrough. Twice daily dosing of PPI may improve the symptoms.

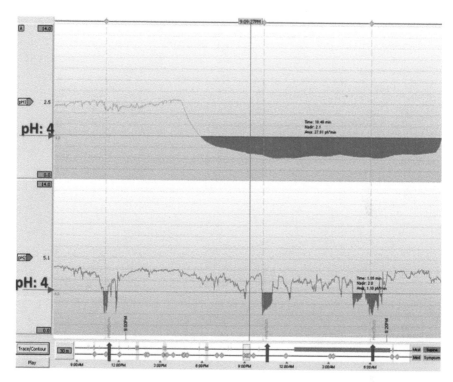

Figure 5.6 pH monitoring with dual pH catheter. The patient had symptoms of heartburn, recurrent sore throat, and globus sensation, suggestive of extraesophageal reflux symptoms. The patient remained "off" acid-suppressive therapy for 5 days before the study. On this tracing, there are two pH sensors. One (*top*) is located distally at 5 cm above the manometrically measured lower esophageal sphincter (LES). The proximal sensor (*bottom*) is 15 cm above the distal sensor. Episodes of acid reflux, as evident by a drop of pH below, are noted in the distal sensor, and the patient recorded three episodes of heartburn associated with this acid reflux (*blue arrows*). More impressively, the proximal sensor detects an extremely long episode of acid reflux, lasting 18 hours. This is certainly not due to proximal extension of the distal acid reflux. With such a prolonged acid reflux episode in the proximal esophagus, one must consider the possibility of an acid-producing inlet patch; further assessment by upper endoscopy is required. When the patient's symptoms are bothersome and/or refractory to PPI, ablation therapy for an inlet patch could be considered

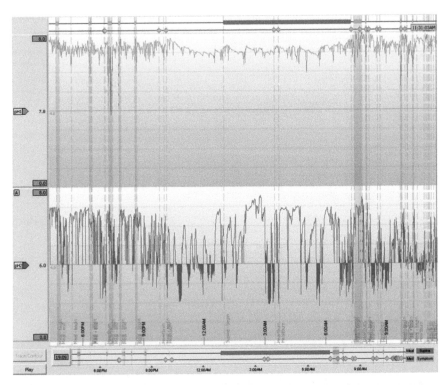

Figure 5.7 24-hour pH monitoring with dual pH catheter in a patient with recurrent heartburn. The study was performed "off" PPI. The patient recorded frequent symptoms, as highlighted at the bottom of the figure. The distal sensor (*bottom*) has detected several episodes of acid reflux, where the pH drops below 4. Some of these episodes are associated with symptoms, but others are not. The acid reflux does not extend proximally; there are no significant acid reflux episodes detected by the proximal sensor (*top*), located 15 cm above the distal pH sensor.

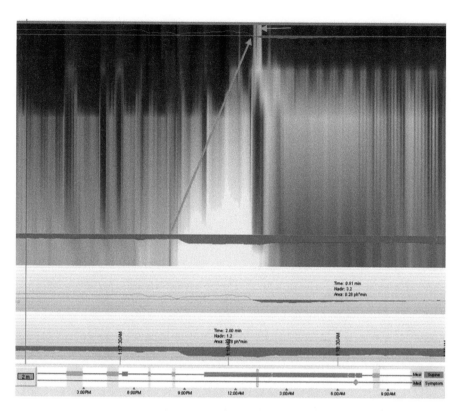

Figure 5.8 24-hour pH monitoring with dual pH-impedance catheter (laryngopharyngeal reflux [LPR] catheter). The catheter has a distal pH sensor, placed 5 cm above the LES, as well as a proximal sensor. The LPR catheter comes in predetermined distances between the proximal and distal pH sensors. The proximal sensor is placed within 1 cm of the manometrically measured upper esophageal sphincter (UES). Therefore, the appropriate catheter length is chosen individually, depending on the distance between the UES and LES, with the consideration of positioning the proximal catheter within 1 cm of the UES. In this figure, the patient has acid reflux, as evident by pH below 4 recorded on the distal sensor. Impedance also shows retrograde liquid refluxate, since there is a drop in impedance. The refluxate extends to the proximal esophagus (*orange arrow*) and is detected by the proximal pH sensor placed at 1 cm above UES (*green arrow*). This finding is highly suggestive of LPR.

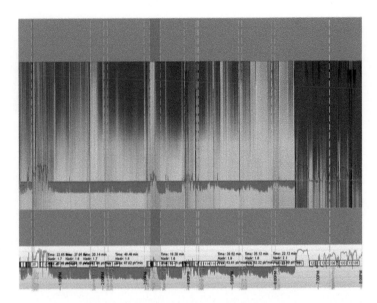

Figure 5.9   24-hour monitoring with pH/ impedance catheter. The distal pH sensor, located 5 cm above the manometrically measured LES, shows a long episode of acid reflux, lasting 5 hours and 30 minutes during the first 6 hours and 30 minutes of the study. Such a prolonged acid reflux duration should raise possible considerations such as a hiatal hernia, slipped or misplaced catheter, or achalasia with food fermentation in the setting of esophageal stasis and incomplete bolus/acidic reflux clearance. Upper endoscopy found that this patient had a large sliding hiatal hernia.

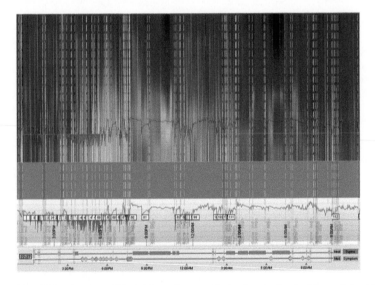

Figure 5.10   pH monitoring with pH-impedance catheter in a patient with persistent GERD symptoms. At the time of this study, the patient was "on" a PPI (dexlansoprazole 60 mg PO QHS). The pH/impedance tracing shows acid breakthrough in the afternoon starting around 3 PM, with recurrent symptoms. There is good correlation of symptoms with episodes of the acid reflux. Based on this study, the patient's PPI dose was increased to BID, which alleviated the symptoms.

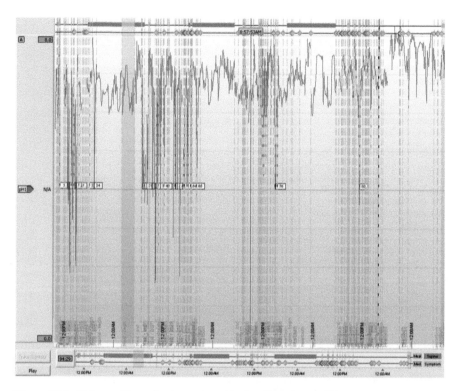

Figure 5.11   96-hour pH monitoring trace with the wireless Bravo™ capsule. The capsule is placed endoscopically 6 cm above the squamocolumnar junction. Note that there is no impedance with the wireless capsule; therefore, the system is incapable of detecting non-acid reflux. However, the system is able to record distal acid exposure for 96 hours, so the test can be split to days "off" PPI (to document pathologic GERD) and days "on" PPI (to assess the patient's response and document a decrease in GERD on medication). In this tracing, the patient was "off" PPI for the first 48 hours, and then resumed PPI. During the first 48 hours, there were episodes of acid reflux, noted by the drop in pH below 4. Acid exposure time at day 1 was 5.6%, day 2 was 3.4%, day 3 was 0.1% and day 4 was 0%. Therefore, the patient has pathologic GERD, which responded well to the PPI.

Figure 5.12 pH-monitoring tracing with a pH/impedance catheter showing aerophagia. Because air increases the resistance to conductivity between two adjacent impedance catheters, the impedance has increased (*asterisks*), hence the darker color on impedance tracing (black/grey). The downward slope of the air movement in the esophagus confirms aboral movement of air in the esophagus. This patient presented with bloating, flatulence, and abdominal distension, secondary to aerophagia.

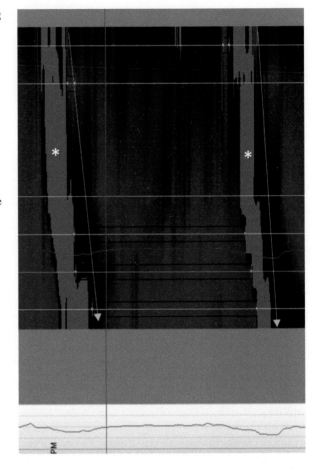

Figure 5.13 pH-monitoring tracing with pH/impedance catheter in a patient with a gastric belch. There is an episode of retrograde refluxate into the distal esophagus (*orange arrow*). The impedance increases (*asterisk*) owing to higher resistance of air to conductivity between the two adjacent impedance sensors. There is likely to be reflux of gastric content in addition to the retrograde gas movement (black/grey), which resulted in the drop in pH, followed by a swallow, outlined as aboral movement of the bolus on impedance (*green arrow*).

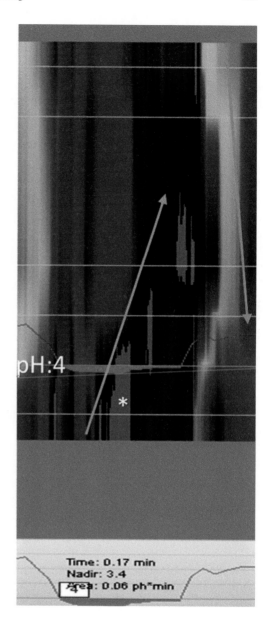

Figure 5.14 pH-monitoring tracing with pH/impedance catheter in a patient with supragastric belch. The gold standard to differentiate gastric from supragastric belching is pH monitoring with impedance. In this tracing, there is an increase in impedance, as evident by darker-colored tracing (*asterisk*). There is aboral movement of air into the proximal esophagus, but shortly afterward, the air moves back up (*orange arrows*). There is no change in pH in the distal esophagus. This is the classic pattern seen in patients with supragastric belch.

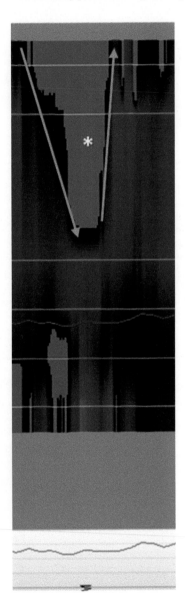

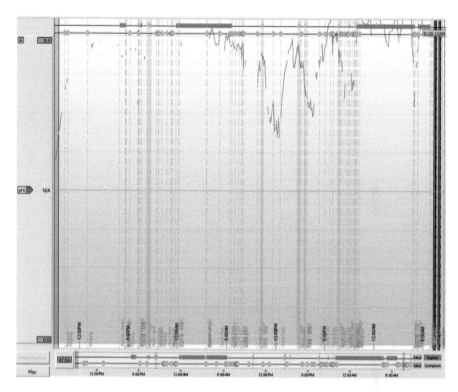

Figure 5.15 48-hour pH monitoring with wireless Bravo™ capsule. The capsule is attached 6 cm proximal to the squamocolumnar junction on upper endoscopy. In this recording, there is frequent interruption in the tracing, which may be due to recorder malfunction, or it could occur if the patient did not keep the recorder in close proximity at all times during the pH evaluation.

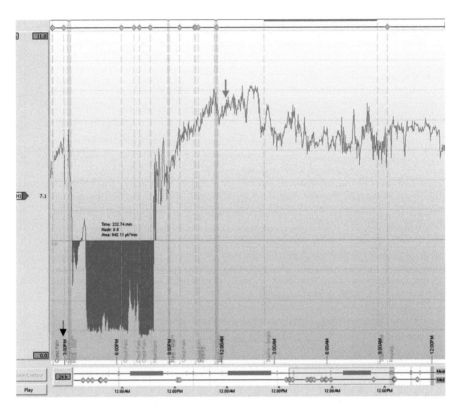

Figure 5.16 pH tracing with wireless Bravo™ capsule. The capsule was placed endoscopically 6 cm above the squamocolumnar junction. The tracing shows an initial episode of acid reflux around 3:00 PM (*black arrow*). Shortly after, the pH recovers to pH above 4. However, the pH declines rapidly, marked by a sharp slope drop to pH of approximately 1 at 4:00 PM. The pH remains as low as 1 for 233 minutes (i.e., gastric transit time), followed by rapid recovery of pH to 6–7 at around 8 PM. The rapid drop in pH is suggestive of Bravo™ capsule dislodgement into the stomach, as gastric pH is as low as 1 with meal onset (also about 3:00 PM). It is common for capsule dislodgment to occur after a meal. At around 8 PM, when the pH recovers to 6–7, the capsule has moved out of the stomach into the small bowel. The capsule probably entered the colon around midnight, as the cecal pH is usually lower than that of small bowel (*green arrow*). Therefore, the small bowel transit time is roughly 6 hours.

References

1. El-Serag HB, Sweet S, Winchester CC, Dent J. Update on the epidemiology of gastro-oesophageal reflux disease: a systematic review. Gut. 2014;63:871–80.
2. Vakil N, van Zanten SV, Kahrilas P, Dent J, Jones R, Global Consensus Group. The Montreal definition and classification of gastroesophageal reflux disease: a global evidence-based consensus. Am J Gastroenterol. 2006;101:1900–20; quiz 1943.
3. Gawron AJ, Pandolfino JE. Ambulatory reflux monitoring in GERD: which test should be performed and should therapy be stopped? Curr Gastroenterol Rep. 2013;15:316.
4. Lacy BE, Chehade R, Crowell MD. A prospective study to compare a symptom-based reflux disease questionnaire to 48-h wireless pH monitoring for the identification of gastroesophageal reflux (revised 2-26-11). Am J Gastroenterol. 2011;106:1604–11.

5. Hirano I, Richter JE, Practice Parameters Committee of the American College of Gastroenterology. ACG practice guidelines: esophageal reflux testing. Am J Gastroenterol. 2007;102:668–85.

6. Gyawali CP, Kahrilas PJ, Savarino E, Zerbib F, Mion F, Smout A, et al. Modern diagnosis of GERD: the Lyon Consensus. Gut. 2018;67:1351–62.

7. Park JM, Kim BJ, Kim JG, Chi KC. Factors predicting outcomes of laparoscopic Nissen fundoplication for gastroesophageal reflux disease: experience at a single institution in Korea. Ann Surg Treat Res. 2017;92:184–90.

8. Katz PO, Gerson LB, Vela MF. Guidelines for the diagnosis and management of gastroesophageal reflux disease. Am J Gastroenterol. 2013;108:308–28; quiz 329.

9. Johnson LF, DeMeester TR. Twenty-four-hour pH monitoring of the distal esophagus. A quantitative measure of gastroesophageal reflux. Am J Gastroenterol. 1974;62:325–32.

10. Sifrim D, Castell D, Dent J, Kahrilas PJ. Gastro-oesophageal reflux monitoring: review and consensus report on detection and definitions of acid, non-acid, and gas reflux. Gut. 2004;53:1024–31.

11. Han MS, Peters JH. Ambulatory esophageal pH monitoring. Gastrointest Endosc Clin N Am. 2014;24:581–94.

12. Jacob P, Kahrilas PJ, Herzon G. Proximal esophageal pH-metry in patients with 'reflux laryngitis'. Gastroenterology. 1991;100:305–10.

13. McCollough M, Jabbar A, Cacchione R, Allen JW, Harrell S, Wo JM. Proximal sensor data from routine dual-sensor esophageal pH monitoring is often inaccurate. Dig Dis Sci. 2004;49:1607–11.

14. Wassenaar E, Johnston N, Merati A, Montenovo M, Petersen R, Tatum R, et al. Pepsin detection in patients with laryngopharyngeal reflux before and after fundoplication. Surg Endosc. 2011;25:3870–6.

15. Hoppo T, Komatsu Y, Jobe BA. Antireflux surgery in patients with chronic cough and abnormal proximal exposure as measured by hypopharyngeal multichannel intraluminal impedance. JAMA Surg. 2013;148:608–15.

16. Shay S, Tutuian R, Sifrim D, Vela M, Wise J, Balaji N, et al. Twenty-four hour ambulatory simultaneous impedance and pH monitoring: a multicenter report of normal values from 60 healthy volunteers. Am J Gastroenterol. 2004;99:1037–43.

17. Zerbib F, Roman S, Bruley Des Varannes S, Gourcerol G, Coffin B, Ropert A, et al. Normal values of pharyngeal and esophageal 24-hour pH impedance in individuals on and off therapy and interobserver reproducibility. Clin Gastroenterol Hepatol. 2013;11:366–72.

18. Borges LF, Chan WW, Carroll TL. Dual pH probes without proximal esophageal and pharyngeal impedance may be deficient in diagnosing LPR. J Voice. 2018; pii: S0892-1997(18)30005-5. [Epub ahead of print].

19. Prakash C, Clouse RE. Value of extended recording time with wireless pH monitoring in evaluating gastroesophageal reflux disease. Clin Gastroenterol Hepatol. 2005;3:329–34.

20. Roman S, Gyawali CP, Savarino E, Yadlapati R, Zerbib F, Wu J, et al. Ambulatory reflux monitoring for diagnosis of gastro-esophageal reflux disease: update of the Porto consensus and recommendations from an international consensus group. Neurogastroenterol Motil. 2017;29:1–15.

21. Vaezi MF, Katzka D, Zerbib F. Extraesophageal symptoms and diseases attributed to GERD: where is the pendulum swinging now? Clin Gastroenterol Hepatol. 2018;16:1018–29.

22. Sifrim D, Dupont L, Blondeau K, Zhang X, Tack J, Janssens J. Weakly acidic reflux in patients with chronic unexplained cough during 24 hour pressure, pH, and impedance monitoring. Gut. 2005;54:449–54.

23. Blondeau K, Dupont LJ, Mertens V, Tack J, Sifrim D. Improved diagnosis of gastro-oesophageal reflux in patients with unexplained chronic cough. Aliment Pharmacol Ther. 2007;25:723–32.

24. Tutuian R, Mainie I, Agrawal A, Adams D, Castell DO. Nonacid reflux in patients with chronic cough on acid-suppressive therapy. Chest. 2006;130:386–91.

25. Patterson N, Mainie I, Rafferty G, McGarvey L, Heaney L, Tutuian R, et al. Nonacid reflux episodes reaching the pharynx are important factors associated with cough. J Clin Gastroenterol. 2009;43:414–9.

26. Ribolsi M, Savarino E, De Bortoli N, Balestrieri P, Furnari M, Martinucci I, et al. Reflux pattern and role of impedance-pH variables in predicting PPI response in patients with suspected GERD-related chronic cough. Aliment Pharmacol Ther. 2014;40:966–73.
27. Aksglaede K, Funch-Jensen P, Thommesen P. Intra-esophageal pH probe movement during eating and talking. A videoradiographic study. Acta Radiol. 2003;44:131–5.
28. Pandolfino JE, Schreiner MA, Lee TJ, Zhang Q, Boniquit C, Kahrilas PJ. Comparison of the Bravo wireless and Digitrapper catheter-based pH monitoring systems for measuring esophageal acid exposure. Am J Gastroenterol. 2005;100:1466–76.
29. Pandolfino JE, Richter JE, Ours T, Guardino JM, Chapman J, Kahrilas PJ. Ambulatory esophageal pH monitoring using a wireless system. Am J Gastroenterol. 2003;98:740–9.
30. Johnson LF, DeMeester TR. Development of the 24-hour intraesophageal pH monitoring composite scoring system. J Clin Gastroenterol. 1986;8(Suppl 1):52–8.
31. Kahrilas PJ, Quigley EM. Clinical esophageal pH recording: a technical review for practice guideline development. Gastroenterology. 1996;110:1982–96.
32. Wang AJ, Wang H, Xu L, Lv NH, He XX, Hong JB, et al. Predictors of clinical response of acid suppression in Chinese patients with gastroesophageal reflux disease. Dig Liver Dis. 2013;45:296–300.
33. de Bortoli N, Martinucci I, Savarino E, Bellini M, Bredenoord AJ, Franchi R, et al. Proton pump inhibitor responders who are not confirmed as GERD patients with impedance and pH monitoring: who are they? Neurogastroenterol Motil. 2014;26:28–35.
34. Patel A, Sayuk GS, Gyawali CP. Parameters on esophageal pH-impedance monitoring that predict outcomes of patients with gastroesophageal reflux disease. Clin Gastroenterol Hepatol. 2015;13:884–91.
35. Patel A, Sayuk GS, Gyawali CP. Acid-based parameters on pH-impedance testing predict symptom improvement with medical management better than impedance parameters. Am J Gastroenterol. 2014;109:836–44.
36. Singh S, Richter JE, Bradley LA, Haile JM. The symptom index. Differential usefulness in suspected acid-related complaints of heartburn and chest pain. Dig Dis Sci. 1993;38:1402–8.
37. Taghavi SA, Ghasedi M, Saberi-Firoozi M, Alizadeh-Naeeni M, Bagheri-Lankarani K, Kaviani MJ, et al. Symptom association probability and symptom sensitivity index: preferable but still suboptimal predictors of response to high dose omeprazole. Gut. 2005;54:1067–71.
38. Kushnir VM, Sathyamurthy A, Drapekin J, Gaddam S, Sayuk GS, Gyawali CP. Assessment of concordance of symptom reflux association tests in ambulatory pH monitoring. Aliment Pharmacol Ther. 2012;35:1080–7.

Index

© Springer Nature Switzerland AG 2020
S. Moosavi et al., *Atlas of High-Resolution Manometry, Impedance, and pH
Monitoring*, https://doi.org/10.1007/978-3-030-27241-8